FIFTH EDITION

Introduction to Audiology

A Review Manual

Frederick N. Martin
The University of Texas at Austin

John Greer Clark
Helix Hearing Care of America

Allyn and Bacon

Boston • London • Toronto • Sydney • Tokyo • Singapore

ISBN 0-205-29537-1

Printed in the United States of America

8   7   6   5   4   3   2   1   03   02   01   00   99

CONTENTS

DISORDERS DESCRIBED IN CASE STUDIES

Acoustic Neuroma
Brainstem Lesion
Central Auditory Lesion
Collapsed Ear Canal
Congenital Hearing Loss
Méniére Disease
Meningitis
Noise-induced Hearing Loss
Nonorganic Hearing Loss—Bilateral
Nonorganic Hearing Loss—Unilateral
Obscure Auditory Dysfunction
Otitis Media
Otosclerosis
Presbycusis
Serous Effusion

PREFACE

The purpose of this book is to help readers to assess their knowledge of the basic concepts of audiology. Previous editions have been used by students in audiology classes, taking comprehensive examinations, or preparing for major tests such as the national examination required of both audiologists and speech language pathologists for certification.

Often students of audiology are not certain that they have learned the important materials from notes and textbooks. This book is designed to allow readers to test their knowledge by completing specific exercises based on facts and concepts that were learned from such sources as textbooks and lectures. There is evidence that learning and reinforcement of learning increase with writing, and so the user of this book is encouraged to fill in the appropriate spaces provided and then check the answers at the end of each unit or chapter. Whenever possible, higher levels of learning are stressed, including application, synthesis, and generalization.

Part I contains fifteen chapters with contents that parallel the seventh edition of *Introduction to Audiology*. Each chapter in this book, like its associated chapter in the text, deals with a specific area of audiology and attempts to utilize a variety of approaches to facilitate learning. In addition, fifteen case studies are provided in Part II, each of which presents a patient's history and some audiometric data. On the basis of this information, the reader should be able to determine the type and degree of hearing loss, discern the probable cause of the disorder, explain why those conclusions were reached, and make recommendations for proper case management.

Although this book is designed as a companion to *Introduction to Audiology*, its use is not necessarily tied to that book. Readers may use other primary sourcebooks or class notes to fill in any missing information. It is of the utmost importance for readers to diagnose their own knowledge deficiencies and correct them in the best and most expeditious way possible, or to enjoy the good feeling that the material has been learned and retained. The following pages will provide further direction on the best ways to use this book.

HOW TO USE THIS BOOK

Part I—Review Chapters

The purpose of this review manual is to assist students in self-identification of strengths and weaknesses in subject mastery. When areas of deficiency are noted, reviewing and learning the material can proceed logically.

This book is not designed to provide new information or to teach new concepts, but rather to assist readers in their efforts to monitor their own grasp of different aspects of audiology. Therefore, the study of each subject should be completed before a given chapter in this book is attempted. If an incorrect answer remains misunderstood, you should return to a primary source for further explanation.

The table of contents lists the fifteen chapters in the book and the fifteen case studies. Some chapters contain more than one unit. Your individual needs and wishes should determine the order in which the chapters are studied.

When you have completed a chapter, check your answers against those at the end of each unit. If you are uncertain of the definitions of some of the terms in the matching exercises, you should review a primary text. The Subject Index in *Introduction to Audiology* can be used to facilitate quick retrieval of the definitions of terms, as those page numbers are printed in *italics*. The greater your working vocabulary, the better your chances of a successful understanding of audiology.

The purpose of the outlines is to help you organize particular subjects. It is more than a mere matching exercise. Of course, if you wish to see the subject organization of a particular chapter without doing the outline, the answers may simply be copied from the back of the unit. The decision on whether to approach the outline with this strategy is left to you.

Part II—Case Studies

Each theoretical case study is three pages long and represents a clinical diagnostic entity. A fourth page is included for notes. Read the history statement on the first page. Then look at the audiogram, tympanogram, and other audiometric data on the second page. After you have reached your conclusions, fill in the appropriate spaces on the first page. Write down the probable etiology (cause) of each hearing disorder. Under "Case Management," write how you would handle the case, to whom a referral might be made, what might be said or written in a report, and so forth. Then write the reasons for your decisions. After this is done, check what you have written against the answers on the third page of the unit.

If more information is required to make a diagnosis, read the appropriate chapter in *Introduction to Audiology* or another textbook. The conditions described in the case studies are listed in alphabetical order in the table of contents, but they are not referred to by page because it is your task to identify the particular disorder from the information provided. Listing the disorders by page numbers would reveal the correct diagnosis ahead of time. You may observe that in the case studies more theoretical test results are presented than are usually obtained in routine practice. This is to illustrate the theoretical findings if all these tests had been performed.

PART I

Review Chapters

1 The Profession of Audiology

Background

Audiology is a young profession with its roots in the development of aural rehabilitation programs designed for servicemen reentering civilian life following World War II. The success of military-based aural rehabilitation programs quickly spurred the development of similar programs within the civilian sector because of the devastating impact of hearing loss on the lives of those affected.

The educational preparation of audiologists grew as its informational and technological bases developed. What began as a bachelor's degree preparation for entering the profession expanded into a required master's degree, and the field is currently evolving into a doctorate-level profession. As audiology has expanded, so has the variety of specialty areas in which audiologists may concentrate; and as the population grows, so does the need for audiological services.

Objectives

1. You should know and understand the terms in the matching exercise.
2. You should be able to fill in the outline, selecting items from the list provided.
3. You should be able to answer the multiple choice questions and recognize the varying responsibilities of audiologists within different specialty areas.

Matching

Match the term from the box on the right with its definition.

Definition

1. _____ The branch of medicine devoted to the study, diagnosis, and treatment of diseases of the ear and related structures

2. _____ The treatment of those with hearing loss that has begun after birth, usually after speech and language development, to improve overall communication ability

3. _____ An organization that adopted the new discipline of audiology in 1947, providing audiology with its first professional home

4. _____ An organization founded in 1988, of, by, and for audiologists

5. _____ The number of existing causes of a disease or disorder in a given population at a given time

Term

a. AAA
b. ASHA
c. Aural rehabilitation
d. Otology
e. Prevalence

Outline

The Profession
Audiology Specialties

1. _____
2. _____
3. _____
4. _____
5. _____

Professional Associations

1. _____
2. _____
3. _____
4. _____
5. _____
6. _____

Select From

A. American Academy of Audiology
B. American Auditory Society
C. Academy of Dispensing Audiologist
D. Academy of Rehabilitative Audiology
E. American Speech-Language-Hearing Association
F. Educational
G. Educational Audiology Association
H. Hearing aid dispensing / Rehabilitative
I. Industrial
J. Medical
K. Pediatric

Multiple Choice

1. At its origin, audiology pooled its knowledge base from
   a. otology
   b. speech pathology
   c. psychology
   d. all of the above
2. The prevalence of hearing loss
   a. decreases over time
   b. increases with age
   c. is unknown
   d. is at an all-time low thanks to modern medical practice
3. The impact of hearing loss
   a. is greater for more severe hearing loss
   b. can affect social maturation
   c. may create an economic burden in excess of one million dollars across an individual's lifetime
   d. all of the above
4. The organization that provided the first "home" for the profession of audiology was
   a. AAS (American Auditory Society)
   b. ARA (Academy of Rehabilitative Audiology)
   c. ASHA (American Speech-Language-Hearing Association)
   d. AAA (American Academy of Audiology)
5. The word "audiology"
   a. means the study of hearing
   b. combines the Latin root, *audire*, with the Greek suffix, *logos*
   c. is often reported to have been coined by the "Father of Audiology," Dr. Raymond Carhart
   d. all of the above

Answers

Matching	*Outline*	*Multiple Choice*

Matching
1. d
2. c
3. b
4. a
5. e

Outline

Audiology Specialties
1. F
2. H
3. I
4. J
5. K

Professional Societies
6. A
7. B
8. C
9. D
10. E
11. G

Multiple Choice
1. d
2. b
3. d
4. c
5. d

2

The Human Ear and Simple Tests of Hearing

UNIT A: THE FUNCTION OF THE EAR

Background

The ear is made up of three portions, the outer ear, the middle ear, and the inner ear. The outer ear is an acoustical chamber that picks up sounds from the environment and resonates at particular frequencies. At the end of the outer ear canal lies the eardrum membrane, which separates the outer ear from the middle ear. The middle ear functions in a primarily mechanical fashion, carrying vibrations to the inner ear via three tiny bones called ossicles. The inner ear is a hydromechanical system that transduces the energy it receives into electrical impulses; these impulses in turn transmit information about sound to the brain by way of the auditory nerve. The auditory system may be divided in a second, different way, one that separates the combined contributions of the outer and middle ears (called the *conductive* mechanism) from those of the inner ear and auditory nerve (the *sensorineural* mechanism). Damage to the conductive mechanism causes a conductive hearing loss, and damage to the sensorineural mechanism causes a sensorineural hearing loss.

Objectives

1. You should know and understand the terms in the matching exercise.
2. You should be able to fill in the outline, selecting items from the list provided.
3. You should be able to label the different parts of the auditory mechanism in Figure 2A.1.
4. You should be able to answer the multiple-choice questions on the function of the ear.

Matching

Match the term from the box on the right with its definition.

Definition

1. _____ The sum of a combination of conductive and sensorineural hearing losses in the same ear

2. _____ Transmission of sound to the inner ear by vibration of the bones of the skull

3. _____ A tone presented to both ears simultaneously is perceived only in the ear in which it is louder

4. _____ Reduction in energy

5. _____ The course of sounds that are conducted to the inner ear by way of the outer and middle ear

6. _____ That portion of the hearing apparatus that converts mechanical energy to electrochemical energy

7. _____ The bony prominence behind the outer ear

8. _____ The most external portion of the hearing mechanism

9. _____ Loss of hearing because of damage to the inner ear or auditory nerve

10. _____ The sense that a sound is in the right or left ear

11. _____ The VIIIth cranial nerve connecting the inner ear with the brain

12. _____ The air-filled cavity behind the eardrum membrane that holds the three smallest bones of the body

13. _____ The loss of sound sensitivity because of damage to the outer or middle ear

14. _____ Reference to the sense of hearing

15. _____ The portion of the inner ear responsible for the hearing function

Term

a. Air conduction
b. Attenuation
c. Auditory
d. Auditory nerve
e. Bone conduction
f. Cochlea
g. Conductive hearing loss
h. Inner ear
i. Lateralization
j. Mastoid process
k. Middle ear
l. Mixed hearing loss
m. Outer ear
n. Sensorineural hearing loss
o. Stenger principle

Outline

The Human Ear
Outer Ear

1. ____
2. ____
3. ____

Middle Ear

4. ____
5. ____
6. ____

Inner Ear

7. ____
8. ____

Auditory Nerve

9. ____

Select From

A. Air-filled space with mucous membrane lining
B. Carries impulses to the brain
C. Eardrum membrane
D. External ear canal
E. Funnel-shaped structure
F. Open air-filled space
G. Snail-like structure
H. Tiniest bones in the body
I. Transducer

Activity

Label the items in Figure 2A.1. Select the terms from the list provided.

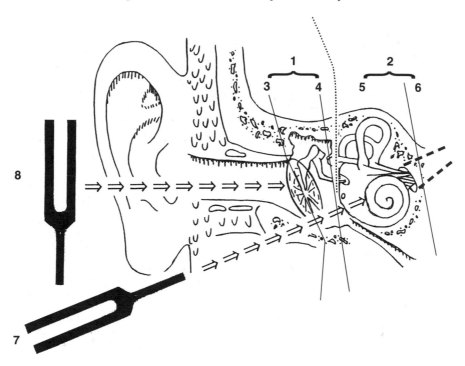

Label		Term
1. _____		**A.** Air-conduction pathway
2. _____		**B.** Auditory nerve
3. _____		**C.** Bone-conduction pathway
4. _____		**D.** Conductive mechanism
5. _____		**E.** Inner ear
6. _____		**F.** Middle ear
7. _____		**G.** Outer ear
8. _____		**H.** Sensorineural mechanism

Multiple Choice

1. The air-conduction pathway is the
   a. outer ear, inner ear, auditory nerve, middle ear
   b. outer ear, middle ear
   c. outer ear, middle ear, inner ear, auditory nerve
   d. inner ear, auditory nerve
2. The bone-conduction pathway is the
   a. outer ear, inner ear, auditory nerve, middle ear
   b. outer ear, middle ear
   c. outer ear, middle ear, inner ear, auditory nerve
   d. inner ear, auditory nerve
3. When air conduction is impaired and bone conduction is normal, the interpretation is
   a. conductive hearing loss
   b. mixed hearing loss
   c. normal hearing
   d. sensorineural hearing loss
4. When air conduction is impaired and bone conduction is impaired to the same degree, the interpretation is
   a. conductive hearing loss
   b. mixed hearing loss
   c. normal hearing
   d. sensorineural hearing loss
5. When air conduction is normal and bone conduction is normal, the interpretation is
   a. conductive hearing loss
   b. mixed hearing loss
   c. normal hearing
   d. sensorineural hearing loss
6. When air conduction is impaired and bone conduction is impaired, but to a lesser degree, the interpretation is
   a. conductive hearing loss
   b. mixed hearing loss
   c. normal hearing
   d. sensorineural hearing loss
7. The conductive mechanism is comprised of
   a. outer ear and middle ear
   b. middle ear and inner ear
   c. inner ear and auditory nerve
   d. auditory nerve and outer ear
8. The sensorineural mechanism is comprised of
   a. outer ear and middle ear
   b. middle ear and inner ear
   c. inner ear and auditory nerve
   d. auditory nerve and outer ear

Answers—Unit A

Matching	*Outline*	*Activity*	*Multiple Choice*
1. l	**1.** D	**1.** D	**1.** c
2. e	**2.** E	**2.** H	**2.** d
3. o	**3.** F	**3.** G	**3.** a
4. b	**4.** A	**4.** F	**4.** d
5. a	**5.** C	**5.** E	**5.** c
6. h	**6.** H	**6.** B	**6.** b
7. j	**7.** G	**7.** C	**7.** a
8. m	**8.** I	**8.** A	**8.** c
9. n	**9.** B		
10. i			
11. d			
12. k			
13. g			
14. c			
15. f			

UNIT B: TUNING FORKS

Background

The tuning fork is a device borrowed from the profession of music by the medical profession. The tuning fork vibrates sinusoidally and comes closer to generating a pure tone than any other nonelectronic device. Most tuning-fork tests were developed by German otologists over a century ago and are still used by many practicing physicians. They have two primary values that justify their study: (1) They are of historical significance, and (2) they illustrate very well the relationships between air conduction (AC) and bone conduction (BC). The Rinne test compares a patient's hearing sensitivity by AC to BC; the Schwabach test compares the patient's hearing by BC to normal (the examiner's) hearing; the Bing test checks for the occlusion effect, which should be absent in conductive hearing losses; the Weber test checks for lateralization in unilateral hearing losses. Tuning-fork tests are non-quantifiable and must be specified in terms of the frequency of the fork being used.

Objectives

1. You should know and understand the terms in the matching exercise.
2. You should be able to fill in the outline, selecting items from the list provided.
3. You should understand the four tuning-fork tests discussed in this unit in terms of performance and interpretation.
4. You should be able to answer the multiple-choice questions and understand the purpose and use of tuning forks.

Matching

Match the term from the box on the right with its definition.

Definition

1. ____ The perception of increased loudness of a bone-conducted tone when the outer ear is occluded

2. ____ A tuning-fork test that compares the patient's hearing sensitivity by bone conduction with the examiner's

3. ____ Sounds that are conducted to the inner ear by vibration of the bones of the skull

4. ____ Attenuation of sounds as they pass through an abnormality of the outer ear or middle ear

5. ____ A metal instrument with a stem and two tines that is designed to vibrate at a single frequency

6. ____ A tone of only one frequency with no overtones

7. ____ A tuning-fork test that checks for the occlusion effect to determine the presence of conductive loss

8. ____ A tuning-fork test that compares hearing sensitivity presented by bone conduction to air conduction

9. ____ Conduction of sound to the inner ear by way of the outer and middle ear

10. ____ A tuning-fork test to determine whether a bone-conducted tone is heard in the right, left, or both ears

11. ____ Hearing loss produced by abnormality of the inner ear or auditory nerve

Term

a. Air conduction
b. Bing test
c. Bone conduction
d. Conductive hearing loss
e. Occlusion effect
f. Pure tone
g. Rinne test
h. Schwabach test
i. Sensorineural hearing loss
j. Tuning fork
k. Weber test

Outline

Tuning Fork Test
Rinne

1. _____
2. _____
3. _____
4. _____
5. _____
6. _____

Schwabach

7. _____
8. _____
9. _____

Bing

10. _____
11. _____
12. _____
13. _____
14. _____

Weber

15. _____
16. _____
17. _____
18. _____

Select From

A. Absence of occlusion effect means conductive hearing loss
B. Compares AC sensitivity to BC
C. Compares patient's BC hearing to examiner's
D. Frequency must be specified
E. Heard in better ear in sensorineural hearing loss
F. Heard in poorer ear in conductive hearing loss
G. Louder by AC means normal or sensorineural loss
H. Louder by BC means conductive loss
I. Presence of OE means normal or sensorineural loss
J. Outer ear is occluded
K. Stem held against forehead
L. Stem held against mastoid
M. Tine held next to ear

Activity

Using Figure 2B.1, indicate the position in which a tuning fork should be held for each test.

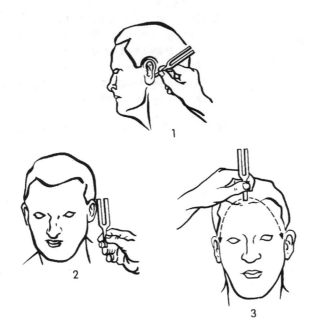

Label		*Term*
1. _____		**A.** Bing test
2. _____		**B.** Rinne test
3. _____		**C.** Schwabach test
		D. Weber test

Multiple Choice

1. One thing that should always be specified when reporting the results of tuning-fork tests is the
   a. frequency of the fork
   b. amplitude of the fork
   c. pressure of the fork against the head
   d. weight of the fork

2. A problem that tuning-fork tests have in common with any measurement made by bone conduction is that
   a. the nontest ear may hear the tone by bone conduction
   b. the patient may feel the vibrations
   c. pressure against the skull is a variable
   d. all of the above

3. In bilateral sensorineural hearing loss, the tuning-fork tests will theoretically show
   a. Bing negative: Rinne negative
   b. Bing positive: Rinne negative
   c. Bing negative: Rinne positive
   d. Bing positive: Rinne positive

4. A patient has a severe sensorineural hearing loss in the left ear and normal hearing in the right ear. Results on the Rinne test would be
   a. left positive: right positive
   b. left false negative: right positive
   c. left negative: right negative
   d. left false negative: right false positive

5. In unilateral conductive hearing loss, the Weber test will result in the sound being heard in the
   a. better ear
   b. both ears
   c. poorer ear
   d. neither ear

6. A normal Schwabach can mean
   a. normal hearing or conductive hearing loss
   b. normal hearing or sensorineural hearing loss
   c. normal hearing or mixed hearing loss
   d. sensorineural hearing loss

The next three questions are based on the proposition that your patient has a moderate conductive hearing loss in the left ear and a moderate sensorineural hearing loss in the right ear.

7. Results on the Rinne test should be
   a. positive right: positive left
   b. negative right: negative left
   c. positive right: negative left
   d. false negative right: negative left

8. If masking is used in the nontest ear, results on the Schwabach should be
   a. normal right: normal left
   b. diminished right: prolonged left
   c. prolonged right: diminished left
   d. normal right: diminished left
9. Results on the Bing test should be
   a. positive right: positive left
   b. negative right: negative left
   c. positive right: negative left
   d. negative right: positive left

Answers—Unit B

Matching	*Outline*	*Activity*	*Multiple Choice*
1. e	**1.** B	**1.** A, B, C	**1.** a
2. h	**2.** D	**2.** B	**2.** d
3. c	**3.** G	**3.** D	**3.** d
4. d	**4.** H		**4.** b
5. j	**5.** L		**5.** c
6. f	**6.** M		**6.** a
7. b	**7.** C		**7.** d
8. g	**8.** D		**8.** b
9. a	**9.** L		**9.** c
10. k	**10.** A		
11. i	**11.** D		
	12. I		
	13. J		
	14. L		
	15. D		
	16. E		
	17. F		
	18. K		

CHAPTER

3   Sound and Its Measurement

Background

Humans are accustomed to hearing sound as a wave disturbance propagated through air. Three properties are necessary to produce sound waves: a force, a vibrating mass, and an elastic medium. Air molecules are the mass undergoing to-and-fro motion (vibration), and air itself has an elastic nature so that the molecules, in their vibratory motion, seem to be connected by "springs." Sound waves are produced by molecular vibration because of the pressure conditions that are created when molecules are packed closer together (compression) or spread further apart (rarefaction) than normal.

As molecules undergo oscillation, successive compressions, followed by rarefactions, are passed along the line of particles at the speed of sound. Waves behaving with simple periodic oscillation are often called sine waves. These waves may be described in terms of how often they move from maximum rarefaction to maximum compression and then return to their point of origin: This is called the frequency of the wave. The intensity of a wave is the force that moves it to its maximum amplitude.

The measurement unit for frequency is cycles per second (cps) or hertz (Hz). The measurement unit for intensity is the decibel (dB), a ratio between two sound pressures or two sound powers. Waves of different frequencies may combine to form interactions called complex waves. Frequency is interpreted psychologically as pitch, and intensity as loudness. Different complex waveforms produce the quality or timbre of a sound.

Objectives

1. You should know and understand the terms in the matching exercise.
2. You should be able to fill in the outline, selecting items from the list provided.
3. You should be able to label the different parts of Figure 3.1 relating to sound waves.
4. You should be able to do the matching exercise on sound measurement units.
5. You should be able to answer the multiple-choice questions on the physics of sound.

Matching 1

Match the term from the box on the right with its definition.

Definition

1. _____ The ability of a mass to return to its natural shape

2. _____ The exponent that tells the power to which a number is raised

3. _____ A unit of power

4. _____ A whole-number multiple of the fundamental of a complex wave

5. _____ The extent of the vibratory movement of a mass to the point furthest from its position of rest

6. _____ The portion of a sound wave where the molecules become less dense

7. _____ The amount of sound energy per unit of area

8. _____ The duration of one cycle of vibration

9. _____ A unit of expressing ratios in base 10 logarithms

10. _____ The waveform of a pure tone showing simple harmonic motion

11. _____ The difference between tones separated by a frequency ratio of 2:1

12. _____ The speed of a sound wave in a given direction

13. _____ A unit of pitch measurement

14. _____ The to-and-fro movements of a mass

15. _____ The distance between the same points on two successive cycles of a tone

16. _____ Reduction in amplitude to zero because of interaction of two tones 180 degrees out of phase

17. _____ The number of complete oscillations of a vibrating body per unit of time

18. _____ A series of moving impulses set up by a vibration

19. _____ Progressive lessening in the amplitude of a vibrating body

Term

a. Amplitude
b. Aperiodic wave
c. Beats
d. Bel
e. Brownian motion
f. Cancellation
g. Component
h. Compression
i. Cosine wave
j. Damping
k. Difference tone
l. Dyne
m. Elasticity
n. Exponent
o. Force
p. Frequency
q. Fundamental frequency
r. Harmonic
s. Intensity
t. Logarithm
u. Mel
v. Microbar
w. Newton
x. Octave
y. Oscillation
z. Overtone
aa. Pascal
ab. Period
ac. Periodic wave
ad. Phase
ae. Phon
af. Rarefaction
ag. Resonance
ah. Sinusoid
ai. Sone
aj. Velocity
ak. Watt
al. Wave
am. Wavelength

Definition

20. _____ The impetus required to increase the velocity of a vibrating body

21. _____ Periodic variations of the amplitude of a tone caused by a second tone of slightly different frequency

22. _____ A unit of pressure equal to 1 Newton per meter square

23. _____ A logarithm

24. _____ A unit of force just sufficient to accelerate a mass of 1 gram at 1 cm per second squared

25 _____ A pressure equal to one-millionth of standard atmospheric pressure

26 _____ The lowest frequency of vibration in a complex wave

27. _____ The frequency of a tone produced by two tones of slightly different frequency

28. _____ A waveform that does not repeat itself over time

29. _____ The relationship in time between two or more waves

30. _____ A force equal to 100,000 dynes

31. _____ The portion of a sound wave where molecules become more dense

32. _____ A pure-tone constituent of a complex wave

33. _____ A unit of loudness measurement

34. _____ A waveform that repeats itself over time

35. _____ The constant colliding movement of molecules in a medium

36. _____ The unit of loudness level

37. _____ The ability of a mass to vibrate at a particular frequency with minimum external force

38. _____ A sound wave representing simple harmonic motion that begins at 90 or 270 degrees

39. _____ Like a harmonic but numbered differently

Term

a. Amplitude
b. Aperiodic wave
c. Beats
d. Bel
e. Brownian motion
f. Cancellation
g. Component
h. Compression
i. Cosine wave
j. Damping
k. Difference tone
l. Dyne
m. Elasticity
n. Exponent
o. Force
p. Frequency
q. Fundamental frequency
r. Harmonic
s. Intensity
t. Logarithm
u. Mel
v. Microbar
w. Newton
x. Octave
y. Oscillation
z. Overtone
aa. Pascal
ab. Period
ac. Periodic wave
ad. Phase
ae. Phon
af. Rarefaction
ag. Resonance
ah. Sinusoid
ai. Sone
aj. Velocity
ak. Watt
al. Wave
am. Wavelength

Outline

Physics of Sound

Waves

1. ____
2. ____
3. ____
4. ____

Vibrations

5. ____
6. ____

Frequency

7. ____
8. ____
9. ____
10. ____

Intensity

11. ____
12. ____
13. ____
14. ____

Decibels

15. ____
16. ____
17. ____

Spectrum

18. ____

Psychological Acoustics

19. ____
20. ____
21. ____

Select From

A. Complex waves
B. Cycles per second
C. Decibel
D. Forced vibration
E. Fourier analysis
F. Free vibration
G. Hearing level
H. Hertz
I. Length effects
J. Longitudinal
K. Loudness
L. Mass effects
M. Pitch
N. Power
O. Pressure
P. Quality
Q. Sensation level
R. Sine
S. Sound-pressure level
T. Transverse
U. Work

Activity

Five parts of the sine wave shown in Figure 3.1 are labeled. Each part may be referred to in two ways. Label each part appropriately.

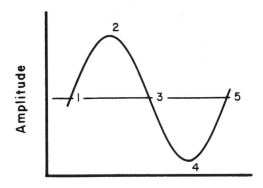

Time/Degrees

FIGURE 3.1   Sine wave.

	Label		**Term**
1.	_____	**A.**	Maximum amplitude
	_____	**B.**	90 degrees
2.	_____	**C.**	180 degrees
	_____	**D.**	360 degrees
3.	_____	**E.**	270 degrees
	_____	**F.**	Zero amplitude
4.	_____	**G.**	0 degees
	_____		
5.	_____		
	_____		

Matching 2

Match the measurement unit to each measurement below.

Measurement

Acceleration

1. ____
2. ____

Area

3. ____
4. ____

Force

5. ____
6. ____

Intensity

7. ____
8. ____

Length

9. ____
10. ____

Mass

11. ____
12. ____

Power

13. ____
14. ____
15. ____

Pressure

16. ____
17. ____
18. ____

Velocity

19. ____
20. ____

Work

21. ____
22. ____

Unit

a. Centimeter (cm)
b. Centimeter per second (cm/s)
c. Centimeter per second squared (cm/s^2)
d. Centimeter squared (cm^2)
e. Dyne (dyn)
f. Dyne per centimeter squared (dyn/cm^2)
g. Erg (e)
h. Ergs per second (e/s)
i. Gram (g)
j. Joule (J)
k. Joules per second (J/S)
l. Kilogram (kg)
m. Meter (m)
n. Meters per second (m/s)
o. Meters per second squared (M/s^2)
p. Meter squared (m^2)
q. Newton (N)
r. Newton per meter squared (N/m^2)
s. Pascal (Pa)
t. Watt (W)
u. Watt per centimeter squared (w/cm^2)
v. Watt per meter squared (w/m^2)

Multiple Choice

1. Sound intensity
   a. decreases linearly as a function of distance from the source
   b. decreases inversely as a function of the square of the distance from the source
   c. is unaffected by the distance from the source
   d. is the same in fluid as in gas
2. Wavelength is
   a. sound velocity divided by frequency
   b. sound frequency divided by velocity
   c. frequency divided by a constant
   d. determined by intensity
3. If the fifth harmonic of a sound is 500 Hz, the fundamental frequency is
   a. indeterminable from the above information
   b. determined by wavelength
   c. 250 Hz
   d. 100 Hz
4. The period of a 100 Hz tone is
   a. 1/1000 sec
   b. 1/100 sec
   c. 1/10 sec
   d. 1 sec
5. Acceleration is
   a. the same as velocity
   b. the same as speed
   c. velocity divided by time
   d. 0 to 60 mph in 9 sec
6. When the expression *sound-pressure level* (*SPL*) is used, this means that the reference is
   a. 10^{-16} watt/cm^2
   b. 0.002 dyn/cm^2
   c. 20 Pascals
   d. 20 micropascals
7. When the expression *intensity level* (*IL*) is used, this means that the reference is not
   a. 10^{-16} watt/cm^2
   b. 10^{-12} watt/m^2
   c. in decibels
   d. 0.0002 dyn/cm^2
8. The unit of measurement for pitch is the
   a. sone
   b. phon
   c. hertz
   d. mel

9. The SPL of a sound with a pressure output of 200 micropascals is
   a. 10 dB
   b. 20 dB
   c. 30 dB
   d. 40 dB
10. The IL of a sound is 50 dB. Its intensity output is
    a. 10^{-7} watt/m^2
    b. 100 dB
    c. 20 micropascals
    d. 0.0002 dyn/cm^2
11. The velocity of sound in air is said to be
    a. 20 mph
    b. 1130 ft/sec
    c. 5286 ft/sec
    d. 14.7 mph
12. Masking may take place when
    a. the masker precedes the signal
    b. the signal precedes the masker
    c. the masker and signal coexist in time
    d. all of the above
13. At its resonant frequency, a mass vibrates
    a. with the least amount of applied energy
    b. with the greatest amount of applied energy
    c. at its least possible amplitude
    d. as a free vibration
14. The condition in which air molecules are packed most tightly together is called the
    a. resonant frequency
    b. rarefaction
    c. sine wave
    d. compression
15. The quality of a sound is also called its
    a. phase
    b. pure tone
    c. timbre
    d. resonance
16. In the propagation of sound, as air molecules are moved further from each other, they are said to be
    a. condensed
    b. compressed
    c. inert
    d. rarefied
17. The log of 1 is
    a. 0
    b. 1
    c. 2
    d. 3

18. Sounds we hear may be the result of
    a. incident waves
    b. reflected waves
    c. composite waves
    d. all of the above
19. The velocity of sound is
    a. unaffected by the medium
    b. greater in denser media
    c. greater in less dense media
    d. none of the above
20. The joule is a unit of
    a. work
    b. power
    c. intensity
    d. frequency
21. The unit of measurement in equal loudness contours is
    a. mel
    b. sone
    c. decibel
    d. phon

Answers

Matching 1	*Outline*	*Activity*
1. m	**1.** A	**1.** F
2. t	**2.** J	G
3. ak	**3.** R	**2.** A
4. r	**4.** T	B
5. a	**5.** D	**3.** C
6. af	**6.** F	F
7. s	**7.** B	**4.** A
8. ab	**8.** H	E
9. d	**9.** I	**5.** D
10. ah	**10.** L	F
11. x	**11.** C	
12. aj	**12.** N	
13. u	**13.** O	
14. y	**14.** U	
15. am	**15.** G	
16. f	**16.** Q	
17. p	**17.** S	
18. al	**18.** E	
19. j	**19.** K	
20. o	**20.** M	
21. c	**21.** P	
22. aa		
23. n		
24. l		
25. v		
26. q		
27. k		
28. b		
29. ad		
30. w		
31. h		
32. g		
33. ai		
34. ac		
35. e		
36. ae		
37. ag		
38. i		
39. z		

Matching 2

1. C
2. O
3. D
4. P
5. E
6. Q
7. U
8. V
9. A
10. M
11. I
12. L
13. H
14. K
15. T
16. F
17. R
18. S
19. B
20. N
21. G
22. J

Multiple Choice

1. b
2. a
3. d
4. b
5. c
6. d
7. d
8. d
9. b
10. a
11. b
12. d
13. a
14. d
15. c
16. d
17. a
18. d
19. b
20. a
21. d

4 Pure-Tone Audiometry

UNIT A: TESTS WITH PURE TONES

Background

The audiogram is a graph that depicts a patient's thresholds of audibility for a series of pure tones. The graph is arranged so that intensity (in dB HL) is shown on the ordinate: the lower on the graph, the greater the intensity, with 0 dB HL near the top and 110 dB HL near the bottom. Frequency is shown on the abscissa: the further to the right, the higher the frequency, with 125 Hz on the left and 8000 Hz on the right. A patient's threshold is measured for each ear by air conduction (AC) with the use of earphones. Threshold is also measured by bone conduction (BC), using a special oscillator. Thresholds are displayed using the appropriate symbol, as shown on a key on the audiogram form. For AC and forehead BC the symbol is placed on the vertical line indicating the frequency tested, where it intersects the horizontal line, showing the intensity required to reach threshold. If forehead BC testing is done, the symbol is placed, in black, adjacent to the vertical line. Red is used for the right ear and blue for the left ear. The AC threshold for each frequency reveals the total amount of hearing loss; the BC threshold reveals the amount of hearing loss (if any) that is sensorineural; the amount by which hearing by AC is poorer than hearing by BC (the air-bone gap [ABG]) reveals the conductive component. AC symbols should be connected with a solid line, and BC symbols may either not be connected or may be connected with a dashed line. Audiograms may show normal hearing, conductive hearing loss, sensorineural hearing loss, or mixed hearing loss.

Objectives

1. You should know and understand the terms in the matching exercise.
2. You should be able to fill in the outline, selecting items from the list provided.
3. You should memorize the symbols used in plotting an audiogram, including those for right and left ear air conduction and bone conduction. You should also know the symbols to use when masking is used in the opposite ear.
4. You should be able to draw an audiogram based on a patient's thresholds for air conduction and bone conduction.
5. You should be able to interpret audiograms in terms of the type and degree of hearing loss.
6. You should be able to answer the multiple-choice questions and understand the purpose and use of the audiogram.

Matching

Match the term from the box on the right with its definition.

Definition

1. ____ The horizontal line on an audiogram or other graph

2. ____ A device for determining the thresholds of hearing

3. ____ The testing of hearing by specially programmed computer-driven audiometers

4. ____ Measurement made of hearing sensitivity by using earphones

5. ____ Failure of a patient to respond to a stimulus that has been heard

6. ____ The average of a patient's thresholds obtained at 500, 1000, and 2000 Hz in each ear

7. ____ The level at which a stimulus is barely perceptible 50 percent of the time

8. ____ Measurement made that tests hearing sensitivity exclusive of the outer and middle ear

9. ____ The amount of sound energy (in decibels) by which the air-conduction threshold exceeds the bone-conduction threshold

10. ____ A graph representing hearing sensitivity (in decibels) as a function of frequency

11. ____ A response during testing when no stimulus has been presented or was presented below the hearing threshold of the subject

12. ____ Testing hearing by having subjects track their own thresholds

13. ____ The vertical line on an audiogram or other graph

Term

a. Abscissa
b. Air-bone gap
c. Air conduction
d. Audiogram
e. Audiometer
f. Békésy audiometry
g. Bone conduction
h. Computerized audiometry
i. Ordinate
j. False negative
k. False positive
l. Pure-tone average
m. Threshold

Outline

Audiogram Interpretation	**Select From**
The Graph	A. AC threshold
Abscissa	B. Blue
1. ____	C. BC threshold
	D. Equal amount of loss for AC and BC
Ordinate	E. 15 dB threshold or lower for AC
2. ____	F. Frequency
3. ____	G. Greater hearing loss by AC, with lesser hearing
4. ____	loss by BC
Code Color	H. Hearing loss by AC, normal hearing by BC
Right Ear	I. Intensity in dB HL
5. ____	J. Red
	K. O (red)
Left Ear	L. Δ (red)
6. ____	M. < (red)
	N. [(red)
Audiogram Types	O. X (blue)
Normal Hearing	P. □ (blue)
7. ____	Q. > (blue)
	R.] (blue)
Audiogram Interpretation	S. ∨ (black)
Conductive Hearing Loss	T. ⌐ (red)
8. ____	U. ⌐ (blue)
Sensorineural Hearing Loss	
9. ____	
Mixed Hearing Loss	
10. ____	
Symbols	
Right Ear AC	
11. ____	
(unmasked)	
12. ____	
(masked)	
Right Ear BC	
13. ____	
(unmasked)	
14. ____	
(masked)	
Left Ear AC	
15. ____	
(unmasked)	
16. ____	
(masked)	

Audiogram Interpretation

Symbols

Left Ear BC

17. ____
(unmasked)

18. ____
(masked)

Forehead BC

19. ____
(unmasked)

20. ____
Right (left ear masked)

21. ____
Left (right ear masked)

Select From

A. AC threshold
B. Blue
C. BC threshold
D. Equal amount of loss for AC and BC
E. 15 dB threshold or lower for AC
F. Frequency
G. Greater hearing loss by AC, with lesser hearing loss by BC
H. Hearing loss by AC, normal hearing by BC
I. Intensity in dB HL
J. Red
K. O (red)
L. Δ (red)
M. < (red)
N. [(red)
O. X (blue)
P. □ (blue)
Q. > (blue)
R.] (blue)
S. ∨ (black)
T. ˥ (red)
U. ˩ (blue)

Activity

Given the four sets of audiometric data below, draw the audiograms that follow (Figures 4A.1 to 4A.4), illustrating four basic conditions. Use the symbol indicating masking when an asterisk (*) is shown. Compare your graphs to the properly drawn audiograms (Figures 4A.5 to 4A.8) at the end of this unit.

TABLE 4A.1 Audiometric Data

	Right Ear						Left Ear					
	250	*500*	*1000*	*2000*	*4000*	*8000*	*250*	*500*	*1000*	*2000*	*4000*	*8000*
AC	40	40	35	40	45	40	35	45	40	40	50	45
BC	−5*	0*	5*	10*	0*	—	0*	0*	5*	5*	0*	—
AC	65	70	70	75	65	75	70	65	70	70	70	75
BC	25*	30*	35*	40*	50*	—	25*	30*	40*	50*	55*	—
AC	0	5	0	5	5	10	5	5	0	−5	0	5
BC	0	0	0	5	5	—	0	5	0	0	0	—
AC	25	30	35	35	50	60	30	40	45	50	60	55
BC	25	35	40	40	55	—	25	35	40	45	55	—

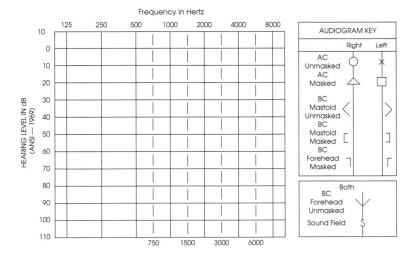

FIGURE 4A.1. Normal hearing.

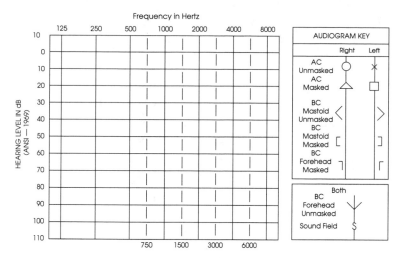

FIGURE 4A.2. Conductive hearing loss.

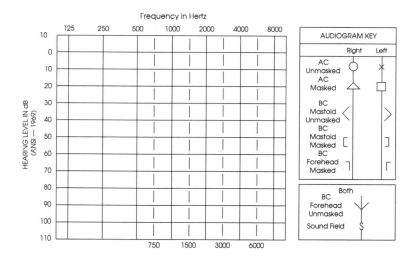

FIGURE 4A.3. Sensorineural hearing loss.

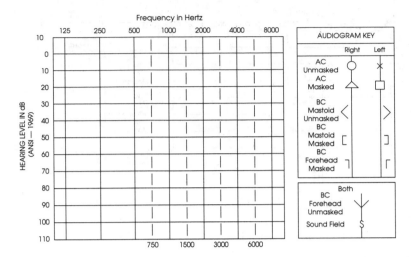

FIGURE 4A.4.   Mixed hearing loss.

Multiple Choice

1. The audiogram showing a conductive type of hearing loss will indicate
   a. impaired bone conduction, normal air conduction
   b. impaired air conduction, normal bone conduction
   c. impaired bone conduction, impaired air conduction
   d. normal bone conduction, normal air conduction
2. The audiogram showing a mixed type of hearing loss will indicate
   a. impaired bone conduction and an air-bone gap
   b. impaired air conduction and no air-bone gap
   c. impaired bone conduction and no air-bone gap
   d. normal bone conduction and an air-bone gap
3. The frequency range for bone conduction on most audiometers is
   a. 125–6000 Hz
   b. 250–8000 Hz
   c. 250–4000 Hz
   d. 125–8000 Hz
4. The maximum testable hearing level for bone conduction on an audiometer is usually
   a. the same as for air conduction
   b. greater than for air conduction
   c. less than for air conduction
   d. both a and c
5. The audiogram showing a sensorineural hearing loss will indicate
   a. impaired bone conduction and an air-bone gap
   b. impaired air conduction and no air-bone gap
   c. impaired bone conduction and normal air conduction
   d. normal bone conduction and an air-bone gap
6. The frequency range for air conduction on most audiometers is
   a. 125–6000 Hz
   b. 250–8000 Hz
   c. 250–4000 Hz
   d. 125–8000 Hz
7. For Figure 4A.4 at 500 Hz, the conductive portion of the hearing loss in the right ear is _____ dB
   a. 70
   b. 30
   c. 40
   d. 35
8. For Figure 4A.3 at 2000 Hz, the conductive portion of the hearing loss in the right ear is _____ dB
   a. 45
   b. 0
   c. –5
   d. 5

9. For Figure 4A.1 at 2000 Hz in the left ear, BC is 5 dB poorer than AC. This suggests
   a. normal variability and may be ignored
   b. a slight conductive hearing loss
   c. a slight sensorineural hearing loss
   d. a slight mixed hearing loss

10. For Figure 4A.2 at 4000 HZ in the left ear, the loss is
    a. completely conductive
    b. completely sensorineural
    c. partially mixed
    d. indeterminable

11. In determining the traditional pure-tone average, the audiometric frequencies used are
    a. 250, 500, 1000 Hz
    b. 1000, 2000, 3000 Hz
    c. 500, 1000, 2000 Hz
    d. 250, 1000, 4000 Hz

12. An apparent sensorineural hearing loss with an air-bone gap only at 3000 and 4000 Hz is probably due to
    a. the occlusion effect
    b. cross-hearing by air conduction
    c. acoustic radiations from the bone-conduction vibrator
    d. acoustic radiations from the air-conduction receiver

13. If an audiogram is properly constructed, the distance across of one octave should be the same as the distance down of
    a. 5 dB
    b. 10 dB
    c. 15 dB
    d. 20 dB

14. Tactile responses to pure tones may be seen when stimuli are
    a. bone conduction only
    b. air conduction only
    c. bone conduction and air conduction
    d. sound field

Answers—Unit A

Matching	*Outline*	*Multiple Choice*
1. a	**1.** I	**1.** b
2. e	**2.** A	**2.** a
3. h	**3.** C	**3.** c
4. c	**4.** F	**4.** c
5. j	**5.** J	**5.** b
6. l	**6.** B	**6.** d
7. m	**7.** E	**7.** c
8. g	**8.** H	**8.** b
9. b	**9.** D	**9.** a
10. d	**10.** G	**10.** a
11. k	**11.** K	**11.** c
12. f	**12.** L	**12.** c
13. i	**13.** M	**13.** d
	14. N	**14.** c
	15. O	
	16. P	
	17. Q	
	18. R	
	19. S	
	20. T	
	21. U	

Activity

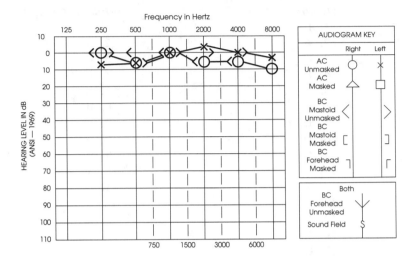

FIGURE 4A.5

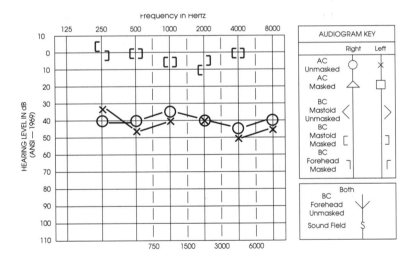

FIGURE 4A.6

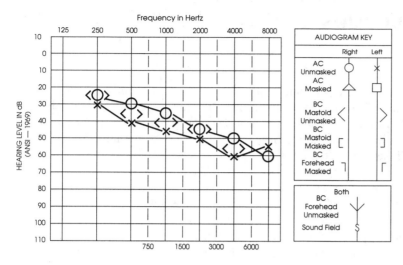

FIGURE 4A.7

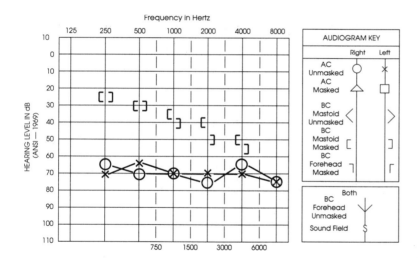

FIGURE 4A.8

UNIT B: BONE CONDUCTION

Background

Bone-conduction tests may be performed with an oscillator from a pure-tone audiometer or the stem of a tuning fork pressed tightly against the skull. Pure-tone bone-conduction audiometry is performed to determine the sensorineural sensitivity of human hearing. Its purpose is to bypass the conductive mechanisms of the outer ear and middle ear and, by distorting the skull, set the structures of the inner ear into vibration, resulting in neural transmission to the brain. The traveling wave set up in the inner ear by bone conduction is intended to stimulate the end organ of hearing. Therefore, whereas air-conduction tests measure the intensity of a signal required to reach a patient's threshold of audibility, including the entire auditory system, bone-conduction tests involve only the sensorineural structures of the inner ear and the pathways beyond. These principles are often violated by certain factors, and in many cases responses to bone conduction stimuli are modified by disorders of the outer ear and middle ear. Because both inner ears are embedded in the bones of the skull, it is virtually impossible to stimulate one without stimulating the other.

Objectives

1. You should know and understand the terms in the matching exercise.
2. You should be able to fill in the outline, selecting items from the list provided.
3. You should understand the principles of bone-conduction tests, why these tests are performed, and why they may not always achieve their objectives.
4. You should be able to answer the multiple-choice questions and grasp the fundamental concepts of bone conduction.

Matching

Match the term from the box on the right with its definition.

Definition

1. _____ The mode of bone conduction involving the middle ear

2. _____ A test of lateralization performed by placing the bone-conduction vibrator on the forehead

3. _____ Introduction of noise into the nontest ear to eliminate cross-hearing

4. _____ The mode of bone conduction involving the outer ear

5. _____ The mode of bone conduction involving only the inner ear

6. _____ The increase in the loudness of bone-conducted tones that occurs when the ear is occluded

7. _____ A device used for calibrating the bone-conduction system of an audiometer

8. _____ Responses to bone-conducted stimuli that have been felt by the patient rather than heard

Term

a. Artificial mastoid
b. Audiometric Weber
c. Distortional
d. Inertial
e. Masking
f. Occlusion effect
g. Osseotympanic
h. Tactile

Outline

Bone Conduction
Outer-ear Effects

1. _____
2. _____

Middle-ear Effects

3. _____
4. _____

Inner-ear Effects

5. _____
6. _____
7. _____
8. _____

Vibrator Placement
Mastoid Advantage

9. _____

Mastoid Disadvantages

10. _____
11. _____
12. _____

Forehead Advantages

13. _____
14. _____

Forehead Disadvantage

15. _____

Air-bone Relationships

16. _____
17. _____

Occlusion Effect

18. _____

Cross Hearing

19. _____
20. _____

Select From

A. Affected by middle-ear conditions
B. Air pressure in middle ear
C. Distortion of temporal bone
D. Effects of covering the ear
E. Energy in outer ear canal
F. Poorer (higher) auditory threshold
G. Improved test reliability
H. Interaural attenuation
I. Intertest variability
J. Less affected by vibrator pressure
K. Better (lower) auditory threshold
L. Masking
M. More affected by vibrator pressure
N. Ossicular chain impedance
O. Oval window release
P. Poor test reliability
Q. Round window release
R. Shearing of hair cells
S. Tactile response
T. Tympanic membrane impedance

Multiple Choice

1. During bone-conduction testing, the low-frequency sounds appear louder when the ear is covered because of
   a. masking
   b. the occlusion effect
   c. the Rinne effect
   d. cross-hearing

2. The mode of bone conduction affected by the outer ear is
   a. osseotympanic
   b. inertial
   c. distortional
   d. compressional

3. Interaural attenuation for bone conduction is generally considered to be _____ dB
   a. 0
   b. 25
   c. 50
   d. 75

4. Intertest variability may cause
   a. AC = BC
   b. AC > BC
   c. AC < BC
   d. all of the above

5. The occlusion effect is found at _____ Hz
   a. 250
   b. 250, 500
   c. 250, 500, 1000
   d. 250, 500, 1000, 2000

6. Testing bone conduction from the forehead requires _____ voltage to produce a response than testing from the mastoid
   a. more
   b. less
   c. the same

7. Forehead placement of the bone-conduction vibrator reduces the _____ mode of bone conduction
   a. inertial
   b. osseotympanic
   c. distortional
   d. compressional

8. The column of air in the external auditory meatus plays a large role in the _____ mode of bone conduction
   a. distortional
   b. osseotympanic
   c. inertial
   d. compressional

9. Advantages of testing bone conduction from the forehead over the mastoid include
   a. less effect of middle-ear disorders
   b. higher intensity required for threshold
   c. lower tactile thresholds
   d. greater interaural attenuation
10. To increase interaural attenuation when masking for bone conduction, one may use
    a. insert receivers
    b. supra-aural receivers
    c. sound field
    d. a hearing aid
11. False air-bone gaps may not be produced by
    a. collapsing ear canals
    b. tactile bone-conduction responses
    c. contralateral bone-conduction responses
    d. distortional bone conduction
12. A profound bilateral sensorineural hearing loss might look like a mixed loss because
    a. cross-hearing is taking place
    b. bone-conduction responses are tactile
    c. ambient noise levels are too high
    d. improper masking is used
13. The mode of bone conduction affected by the inner ear is
    a. fractional
    b. unknown
    c. distortional
    d. osseotympanic
14. The impedance of the ossicular chain plays an important role in the ____ mode of bone conduction
    a. osseotympanic
    b. distortional
    c. inertial
    d. compressional
15. As frequency increases, the occlusion effect
    a. decreases
    b. increases
    c. remains unchanged
    d. decreases, then increases
16. In testing by bone conduction with the vibrator on the right mastoid process, the sound may be heard in
    a. the right ear
    b. the left ear
    c. both ears
    d. all of the above

Answers—Unit B

Matching	*Outline*	*Multiple Choice*
1. d	**1.** E	**1.** b
2. b	**2.** T	**2.** a
3. e	**3.** N	**3.** a
4. g	**4.** B	**4.** d
5. c	**5.** C	**5.** c
6. f	**6.** R	**6.** a
7. a	**7.** O	**7.** a
8. h	**8.** Q	**8.** b
	9. K	**9.** a
	10. P	**10.** a
	11. A	**11.** d
	12. M	**12.** b
	13. G	**13.** c
	14. J	**14.** c
	15. F	**15.** a
	16. I	**16.** d
	17. S	
	18. D	
	19. H	
	20. L	

UNIT C: MASKING

Background

Masking may be defined as the elevation of the threshold of a signal produced by a second, concurrent signal. The signal that is masked is called the maskee, and the signal that elevates the threshold is called the masker. In pure-tone audiometry the maskee is a pure tone and the masker is a noise. The noise should be specified in terms of its spectrum and its effectiveness in producing a threshold shift. Unless audiologists understand the effectiveness of the masking noise they use, they can do little more than work in the dark. Clinical masking must be applied whenever there is a danger that a signal presented to the test ear may reach the threshold of the nontest ear by cross-hearing. Cross-hearing for air conduction (AC) is generally considered to occur primarily by bone conduction (BC). The loss of intensity of a signal as it travels from the test ear earphone to the cochlea of the nontest ear is called interaural attenuation (IA). IA averages from 50–65 dB for supra-aural receivers and from 65 to 100 dB for insert receivers. IA varies with different people and with frequency but has not been reported to be less than 40 dB for supra-aural phones or 65 dB for inserts. These are conservative values to use when deciding on the need to mask. Since BC oscillations vibrate both cochleas with essentially equal force, the IA for BC is considered to be 0 dB. Masking for BC tests may be carried out in every case, but must be implemented when masking might make a difference in diagnosis, that is, when there is an air-bone gap (ABG) in the test ear greater than 10 dB. If cross-hearing has taken place, the only way the threshold of the test ear can be determined is by the plateau method.

Objectives

1. You should know and understand the terms in the matching exercise.
2. You should be able to fill in the outline, selecting items from the list provided.
3. Based on the audiogram in Figure 4C.1, you should be able to determine the need to mask for each frequency for air conduction and bone conduction.
4. You should be able to determine the minimum amount of noise required to just mask out the nontest ear, when necessary.
5. You should be able to label the parts of the masking plateau model in Figure 4C.2.
6. You should be able to answer the multiple-choice questions and grasp the fundamental concepts of masking.

Matching

Match the term from the box on the right with its definition.

Definition

1. _____ A broadband noise containing approximately equal energy per cycle

2. _____ The level of noise that can be varied over a small range that does not alter the threshold of a sound presented to the opposite ear

3. _____ Introduction of noise into the nontest ear to eliminate cross-hearing

4. _____ The hearing of a sound in the ear opposite the one being tested

5. _____ The loss of energy of a sound as it travels from the test ear to the non-test ear

6. _____ A slight shift in threshold of a signal produced by a signal presented to the opposite ear that is not caused by peripheral (crossed) masking

7. _____ A band of frequencies surrounding a pure tone that is just wide enough to produce a threshold shift

8. _____ Masking of a stimulus produced by a noise in the nontest ear that crosses the skull and shifts the threshold of the test ear

9. _____ The lowest level of effective masking presented to the nontest ear during audiometry

10. _____ A broadband masking noise with energy concentrated in the low fre-quencies

11. _____ A system for calibrating a masking signal for simple operation of clini-cal masking procedures

12. _____ A restricted band of frequencies surrounding a particular frequency to be masked

Term
a. Central masking
b. Complex noise
c. Critical band
d. Cross hearing
e. Effective masking
f. Initial masking
g. Interaural attenuation
h. Masking
i. Maximum masking
j. Narrowband noise
k. Overmasking
l. Plateau
m. Undermasking
n. White noise

Definition

13. _____ The highest level of noise that can be presented to one ear before it crosses the skull and masks the opposite ear

14. _____ The result of insufficient noise presented to the nontest ear so that the threshold of the test ear cannot be determined

Term

a. Central masking
b. Complex noise
c. Critical band
d. Cross hearing
e. Effective masking
f. Initial masking
g. Interaural attenuation
h. Masking
i. Maximum masking
j. Narrowband noise
k. Overmasking
l. Plateau
m. Undermasking
n. White noise

Outline

Masking for Pure Tones

The Need to Mask

For AC

1. _____

For BC

2. _____
3. _____

Interaural Attenuation

For AC

4. _____

For BC

5. _____

The Plateau Components

6. _____
7. _____
8. _____
9. _____
10. _____

Noise Types

11. _____
12. _____
13. _____
14. _____
15. _____

Occlusion Effect—Frequencies

16. _____
17. _____
18. _____

Select From

A. ABG greater than 10 dB in test ear
B. $AC_{TE} - IA \geq BC_{NTE}$
C. Average 55 dB (minimum 40 dB) for supra-aural receivers; average 85 dB (minimum 65 dB) for inserts
D. Broadband
E. Complex
F. In all cases
G. Maximum masking
H. Minimum masking
I. Narrowband
J. Overmasking
K. Pink
L. Plateau
M. Sawtooth
N. Undermasking
O. 0 dB
P. 250 Hz
Q. 500 Hz
R. 1000 Hz

Activity

In Table 4C.1 indicate in the proper box whether masking is needed and the minimum amount of effective masking required to mask the nontest ear.

TABLE 4C.1   Masking for an Audiogram

	Tone Right (Masking Left)			
	AC		BC	
Frequency (Hz)	Masking needed?	Min EM	Masking needed?	Min EM
250				
500				
1000				
2000				
4000				
	Tone Left (Masking Right)			
250				
500				
1000				
2000				
4000				

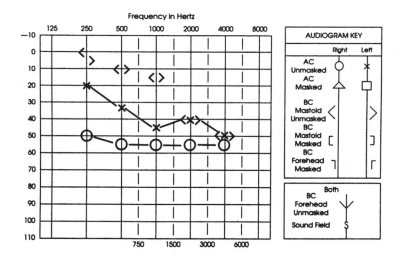

FIGURE 4C.1   An unmasked audiogram.

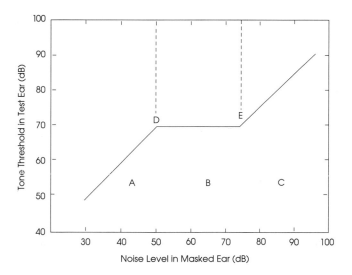

FIGURE 4C.2   A plateau model.

Label the five components of the plateau model.

A. _____

B. _____

C. _____

D. _____

E. _____

Multiple Choice

1. Cross-hearing is a possibility during pure-tone air conduction tests when
   a. $SRT_{TE} - 35 \text{ dB} = BC_{NTE}$
   b. $ABG > 10 \text{ dB}$
   c. $AC_{TE} - IA > BC_{NTE}$
   d. $AC_{TE} - BC_{NTE} = ABG$
2. The primary way by which cross-hearing for air conduction takes place is by
   a. skin conduction
   b. air conduction
   c. bone conduction
   d. cartilage conduction
3. The energy lost as sound travels from one ear to the other is called
   a. interaural attenuation
   b. cross-hearing
   c. contralateralization
   d. lateralization
4. The occlusion effect is tested during the _____ test.
   a. Bing
   b. Rinne
   c. Schwabach
   d. Weber
5. Minimum masking for bone conduction at 250 Hz is
   a. $EM = AC_{TE} + OE$
   b. $EM = AC_{NTE} + OE$
   c. $EM = AC_{TE} - IA$
   d. $EM = AC_{NTE} - IA$
6. Unmasked results on a patient with one normal ear and one ear with a total sensorineural loss show the poorer ear to have
   a. moderate conductive hearing loss
   b. moderate sensorineural hearing loss
   c. profound conductive hearing loss
   d. normal hearing
7. The audiometric Bing test determines the need for additional masking for
   a. bone conduction
   b. word recognition
   c. air conduction
   d. SRT
8. A predicted loss of sensitivity to an auditory stimulus in the presence of contralateral noise is called
   a. overmasking
   b. undermasking
   c. initial masking
   d. central masking

9. Masking is indicated for bone conduction when
   a. $ABG_{TE} > 10$ dB
   b. $ABG_{NTE} > 10$ dB
   c. $BC_{TE} - BC_{NTE} > 10$ dB
   d. $AC > 40$ dB
10. Overmasking is the greatest problem in
    a. bilateral conductive loss
    b. unilateral conductive loss
    c. bilateral sensorineural loss
    d. unilateral sensorineural loss
11. The most efficient kind of masking noise for pure-tone testing is
    a. narrowband noise
    b. broadband noise
    c. high-pass filtered noise
    d. pink noise
12. The masking plateau becomes narrower as the
    a. BC threshold in the test ear gets lower (better)
    b. BC threshold in the test ear gets higher (poorer)
    c. interaural attenuation gets greater
    d. AC threshold in the test ear gets lower (better)
13. As the interaural attenuation increases, the masking plateau
    a. stays the same
    b. gets narrower
    c. gets wider
    d. changes in midfrequencies
14. Overmasking takes place for air conduction when
    a. $BC_{TE} + IA = EM_{NTE}$
    b. $BC_{TE} + IA - 10$ dB $= EM_{NTE}$
    c. $EM_{NTE} - ABG_{NTE} < $ True AC_{TE}
    d. $EM_{NTE} - ABG_{NTE} = $ True AC_{TE}

Answers—Unit C

Matching				*Outline*				*Activity*	*Multiple Choice*	

Matching

1. n **8.** k
2. l **9.** f
3. h **10.** b
4. d **11.** e
5. g **12.** j
6. a **13.** i
7. c **14.** m

Outline

1. B **10.** N
2. A **11.** D
3. F **12.** E
4. C **13.** I
5. O **14.** K
6. G **15.** M
7. H **16.** P
8. J **17.** Q
9. L **18.** R

Activity

Plateau

A. Undermasking
B. Plateau (range of EM in decibels)
C. Overmasking
D. Minimum masking
E. Maximum masking

Multiple Choice

1. c **8.** d
2. c **9.** a
3. a **10.** a
4. a **11.** a
5. b **12.** a
6. a **13.** c
7. a **14.** a

TABLE 4C.2 Audiometric Results with Masking

Tone Right
(Masking Left)

Frequency (Hz)	AC		BC	
	Masking needed?	Min EM	Masking needed?	Min EM
250	yes	20	yes	20 + OE
500	yes	35	yes	35 + OE
1000	yes	45	yes	45 + OE
2000	no	—	yes	40
4000	no	—	no	—

Tone Left
(Masking Right)

Frequency (Hz)	AC		BC	
	Masking needed?	Min EM	Masking needed?	Min EM
250	no	—	yes	50 + OE
500	no	—	yes	55 + OE
1000	no	—	yes	55 + OE
2000	no	—	no	—
4000	no	—	no	—

5 Speech Audiometry

UNIT A: SPEECH-HEARING TESTS

Background

Speech audiometry takes several forms and serves a number of useful purposes. Speech may be delivered by monitored live voice or tape or disk recording to a patient via earphones or loudspeakers. Measurements can be made of a patient's threshold of audibility, word recognition, and most comfortable and uncomfortable listening levels. Speech audiometry is helpful in the diagnosis of the type and degree of hearing impairment, in the location of site of lesion, in rehabilitative measures such as assessment of hearing aids, and in determining the reliability of other tests like the pure-tone audiogram.

Objectives

1. You should know and understand the terms in the matching exercise.
2. You should be able to fill in the outline, selecting items from the list provided.
3. You should be able to label the different parts of Figure 5A.1, showing the performance-intensity functions of speech stimuli.
4. You should be able to predict, within reason, speech test results from an audiogram.
5. You should be able to answer the multiple-choice questions and understand the uses and interpretations of speech audiometry.

Matching

Match the term from the box on the right with its definition.

Definition

1. _____ The SPL at which speech becomes uncomfortably loud

2. _____ Introduction of speech through a microphone during speech audiometry

3. _____ A closed-message word-recognition test with emphasis on unvoiced consonants

4. _____ The highest word-recognition score obtainable from an individual regardless of sensation level

5. _____ The lowest level at which an individual can detect the presence of speech and recognize it as speech

6. _____ Monosyllabic words containing three phonemes each that are used in word-recognition tests

7. _____ A short phrase that precedes the stimulus word during speech audiometry

8. _____ A test that uses pictures to determine word recognition scores for children

9. _____ The difference (in decibels) between the threshold for speech and the level at which speech becomes uncomfortably loud

10. _____ Rapidly delivered, monotonous, and unemotional speech

11. _____ A device used for measurement of speech recognition thresholds and word-recognition scores

12. _____ A two-syllable word, used in speech audiometry, that has equal stress on both syllables

13. _____ A graph showing the percentage correct on word-recognition tests as a function of intensity

Term

a. California consonant test
b. Carrier phrase
c. Cold running speech
d. CNC words
e. Diagnostic audiometer
f. Monitored live voice
g. Most comfortable loudness
h. PB max
i. PI/PB function
j. PB word list
k. Range of comfortable loudness
l. Rhyme test
m. Rollover ratio
n. Speech-detection threshold
o. Speech-recognition threshold
p. Spondaic word
q. Uncomfortable loudness level
r. WIPI test

Definition

14. _____ A list of monosyllabic words used for determination of word-recognition scores

15. _____ PB Max – PB Min/PB Max

16. _____ The lowest intensity at which 50 percent of a list of spondees can be recognized

17. _____ The intensity (in dB HL) at which speech is judged to be most comfortably loud

18. _____ A closed-set word recognition test

Term

a. California consonant test
b. Carrier phrase
c. Cold running speech
d. CNC words
e. Diagnostic audiometer
f. Monitored live voice
g. Most comfortable loudness
h. PB max
i. PI/PB function
j. PB word list
k. Range of comfortable loudness
l. Rhyme test
m. Rollover ratio
n. Speech-detection threshold
o. Speech-recognition threshold
p. Spondaic word
q. Uncomfortable loudness level
r. WIPI test

Outline

Speech Audiometry

Speech-Detection Threshold
Purpose
1. _____

Material
2. _____

Speech-Recognition Threshold
Purposes
3. _____
4. _____
5. _____
6. _____

Materials
7. _____
8. _____

Word-Recognition Scores
Purposes
9. _____
10. _____
11. _____

Materials
12. _____
13. _____
14. _____
15. _____
16. _____
17. _____
18. _____

Most Comfortable Loudness
Purpose
19. _____

Material
20. _____

Uncomfortable Loudness
Purpose
21. _____

Material
22. _____

Select From

A. CNC words
B. California Consonant Test
C. Cold running speech
D. Degree of hearing loss for speech
E. Detect presence of speech
F. Intensity of greatest ease of listening
G. Intensity at which speech is just too loud
H. PB word lists
I. Reference level for WRS
J. Rhyme tests
K. Sentence tests
L. Site-of-lesion diagnosis
M. Spondaic words
N. Synthetic sentence identification
O. Verify audiogram
P. Verify hearing aids' benefit
Q. WIPI test
R. Word recognition ability
S. 50 percent discrimination of speech

Activity

Label the four curves shown in Figure 5A.1 that illustrate performance intensity functions. Select the terms from the list provided.

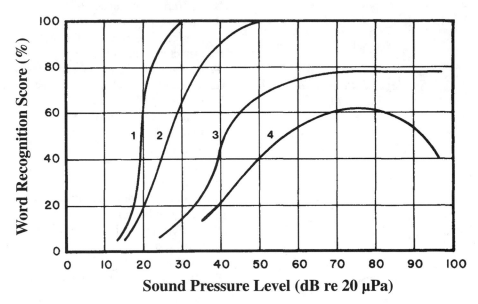

FIGURE 5A.1.   Performance-intensity functions.

Label		*Term*
1. _____		**A.** Normal PB curve
2. _____		**B.** Normal spondee curve
3. _____		**C.** Rollover
4. _____		**D.** Word-recognition loss

Multiple Choice

Answer questions 1–7 based on the information contained in the audiogram in Figure 5A.2. If you are uncertain of the answer to question 1, check the answer at the end of this unit before proceeding with the questions.

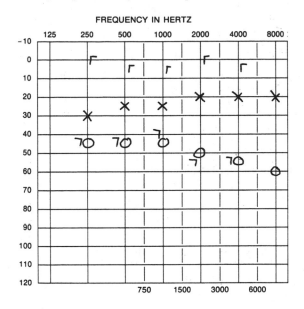

FIGURE 5A.2. An audiogram.

1. The audiogram illustrates
   a. left mild conductive, right moderate conductive
   b. left mild sensorineural, right moderate sensorineural
   c. left mild conductive, right moderate sensorineural
   d. left moderate sensorineural, right mild conductive
2. A predicted SRT for the left ear is _____ dB HL
   a. 5
   b. 25
   c. 45
   d. 70
3. A predicted WRS for the left ear is _____ percent
   a. 6
   b. 40
   c. 80
   d. 100

4. A predicted MCL for the right ear is _____ dB HL
   a. 10
   b. 30
   c. 50
   d. 80
5. A predicted WRS for the right ear is _____ percent
   a. 10
   b. 30
   c. 80
   d. 100
6. A predicted UCL for the left ear is ___ dB HL
   a. 5
   b. 65
   c. 80
   d. 110
7. A predicted RCL (dynamic range) for the right ear is _____ dB
   a. 0
   b. 15
   c. 45
   d. 110
8. The relationship between SRT and SDT is usually
   a. SRT 10 dB lower (better) than SDT
   b. SRT 10 dB higher (poorer) than SDT
   c. SRT the same as SDT
   d. no relationship exists
9. Word-recognition scores are most commonly determined by using
   a. spondees
   b. PB word lists
   c. cold running speech
   d. WIPI
10. SRTs are usually measured with
    a. PB word lists
    b. spondaic words
    c. rhyming words
    d. nonsense words
11. The PI function for spondees is usually
    a. the same as for PBs
    b. more gradual than for PBs
    c. steeper than for PBs
    d. unreliable above 80 dB HL
12. The last word of the carrier phrase in word-recognition testing with PB word lists
    should
    a. strike zero on the volume units (VU) meter
    b. be equal in energy to the PB word
    c. be less intense than the PB word
    d. be more intense than the PB word

13. In audiograms showing sharply falling (in the higher frequencies) sensorineural hearing loss, the SRT is best predicted by the average of the thresholds at _____ Hz
    a. 500 and 1000
    b. 500, 1000, and 2000
    c. 500, 1000, 2000, and 3000
    d. 500, 1000, 2000, 3000, and 4000
14. The word-recognition score expected of a patient with a mild cochlear hearing loss is _____ percent
    a. 0
    b. 50
    c. 80
    d. 100
15. The word-recognition score expected of a patient with moderate conductive hearing loss is _____ percent
    a. 0
    b. 50
    c. 70
    d. 100
16. RCL(DR) is determined by the difference (in decibels) between
    a. UCL and SRT
    b. UCL and MCL
    c. MCL and SRT
    d. UCL and PTA
17. The slope of the normal PI-PB function averages _____ percent per dB
    a. 2.5
    b. 5
    c. 10
    d. 12.5
18. PB MAX – PB MIN/PB MAX is the formula for
    a. percentage of hearing impairment
    b. rollover ratio
    c. word recognition score
    d. none of the above

Answers—Unit A

Matching	*Outline*	*Activity*	*Multiple Choice*
1. q	**1.** E	**1.** B	**1.** c
2. f	**2.** C	**2.** A	**2.** b
3. a	**3.** D	**3.** D	**3.** d
4. h	**4.** S	**4.** C	**4.** d
5. n	**5.** I		**5.** c
6. d	**6.** O		**6.** d
7. b	**7.** C		**7.** c
8. r	**8.** M		**8.** b
9. k	**9.** R		**9.** b
10. c	**10.** P		**10.** b
11. e	**11.** L		**11.** c
12. p	**12.** A		**12.** a
13. i	**13.** B		**13.** a
14. j	**14.** H		**14.** c
15. m	**15.** J		**15.** d
16. o	**16.** K		**16.** a
17. k	**17.** N		**17.** a
	18. Q		**18.** b
	19. F		
	20. C		
	21. G		
	22. C		

UNIT B: MASKING

Background

The possibility of cross-hearing during pure-tone tests is determined by comparing the air-conduction threshold of the test ear to the bone-conduction threshold of the nontest ear at the same frequency. This is done frequency by frequency. If the difference exceeds what may be the interaural attenuation for a given frequency, retesting must be done with masking in the nontest ear. The possibility of cross-hearing during speech audiometry is more difficult to determine because the level of this complex broadband signal (speech) presented by air conduction to one ear must be compared to a pure-tone threshold obtained by bone conduction in the opposite ear. Since it cannot be known which of the frequencies in the nontest ear may contribute to cross-hearing of a speech signal, it is safest to compare to the lowest bone-conduction threshold at any frequency, although frequencies below 500 Hz probably contribute very little to the discrimination of speech. When the difference exceeds a conservative figure set for interaural attenuation (40 dB for supra-aural earphones, 70 dB for insert earphones), masking should be applied to the nontest ear to render it temporarily incapable of responding. The use of effective masking (EM) appears to be the simplest way of approaching masking during speech recognition threshold and word-recognition testing. The problem of overmasking is greatest during word-recognition testing when there is a hearing loss in the masked ear (requiring a higher level of noise) and an air-bone gap in the test ear.

Objectives

1. You should know and understand the terms in the matching exercise.
2. You should be able to fill in the outline, selecting items from the list provided.
3. You should be able to determine the need to mask, based on an audiogram and unmasked SRTs.
4. You should be able to determine the minimum amount of effective masking noise required to just mask out the nontest ear when necessary.
5. You should be able to determine when overmasking has taken place.
6. You should be able to answer the multiple-choice questions and grasp the fundamental concepts of masking for speech audiometry.

Matching

Match the term from the box on the right with its definition.

Definition

1. _____ The ear opposite the one being tested

2. _____ The loss of energy of a (speech) sound as it travels from one ear to the other

3. _____ The lowest intensity at which approximately 50 percent of a group of spondees can be identified correctly

4. _____ The difference (in decibels) between the air-conduction and bone-conduction thresholds

5. _____ Insufficient noise to eliminate the nontest ear from participation in a speech test

6. _____ The greatest amount of noise that can be delivered to the nontest ear without overmasking

7. _____ The act of the nontest ear hearing a speech signal that is presented to the test ear

8. _____ A noise level high enough to lateralize from the nontest ear to the test ear and shift the threshold of the test ear

9. _____ The percentage of correctly identified items on a word-recognition test

10. _____ The least amount of noise required to barely mask out a signal in the same ear

11. _____ The ear being examined on a hearing test

12. _____ The intensity at which a noise can be elevated three times without affecting the audibility of a speech signal in the test ear

13. _____ A reasonable system for calibration of a masking noise

Term

a. Air-bone gap
b. Cross-hearing
c. Effective masking
d. Interaural attenuation
e. Masking
f. Maximum masking
g. Minimum masking
h. Nontest ear
i. Overmasking
j. PB hearing level
k. Plateau
l. Speech-recognition threshold
m. Test ear
n. Undermasking
o. Word-recognition score

Definition

14. _____ The elevation of the threshold of a signal produced by the introduction of a second signal

15. _____ The hearing level at which an audiometer is set to carry out word-recognition testing with PB word lists

Term

a. Air-bone gap
b. Cross-hearing
c. Effective masking
d. Interaural attenuation
e. Masking
f. Maximum masking
g. Minimum masking
h. Nontest ear
i. Overmasking
j. PB hearing level
k. Plateau
l. Speech-recognition threshold
m. Test ear
n. Undermasking
o. Word-recognition score

Outline

Masking for Speech Tests
The Need to Mask
For SRT

1. _____

For WRS

2. _____

Interaural Attenuation

3. _____
4. _____

Minimum EM for SRT

5. _____

Minimum EM for WRS

6. _____

Noise Type

7. _____

Select From

A. Average 55 dB for supra-aural phones, 90 dB for insert phones
B. Broadband
C. Equal to SRT of NTE
D. Minimum 40 dB for supra-aural phones, 90 dB for insert phones
E. $PBHL_{TE} - IA + ABG_{NTE}$
F. $PBHL_{TE} - IA \geq$ lowest BC_{NTE}
G. $SRT_{TE} - IA \geq$ lowest BC_{NTE} (not including 250 Hz)

Activity

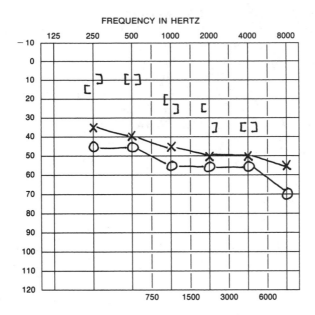

In Table 5B.1, indicate in the proper box whether masking is needed for SRT and word-recognition testing for each ear; also indicate the minimum amount of effective masking required to mask the nontest ear (if necessary). Assume that the word-recognition test is done at 35 dB above the SRT and supra-aural earphones are used.

TABLE 5B.1   Chart for Masking

	Speech Right **(Masking Left)**			**Speech Left** **(Masking Right)**	
Test	*Masking needed?*	*Min EM*	*Test*	*Masking needed?*	*Min EM*
SRT-55 dB			SRT-45 db		
WRS-?%			WRS-?%		

Multiple Choice

1. Of the following the most efficient masker to use during speech audiometry is
   a. narrowband noise
   b. broadband noise
   c. pure tone
   d. the identical signal presented to the test ear

2. It is always necessary to mask for word-recognition testing when
   a. there is an air-bone gap in the test ear greater than 25 dB
   b. the patient's interaural attenuation exceeds 30 dB
   c. the audiograms are asymmetrical
   d. masking was needed for SRT testing

3. The interaural attenuation for speech can be determined if
   a. there is an air-bone gap in the test ear
   b. the unmasked SRT is obtained by cross-hearing
   c. the test ear has a conductive hearing loss
   d. the test ear has a sensorineural hearing loss

4. For word-recognition tests, overmasking creates the greatest problem in
   a. bilateral mixed loss
   b. unilateral mixed loss
   c. bilateral sensorineural loss
   d. unilateral sensorineural loss

5. The need to mask during SRT testing is determined by comparing the
   a. SRT of the test ear to the pure-tone average of the nontest ear
   b. SRT of the test ear to the SRT of the nontest ear
   c. unmasked SRT to the opposite ear bone-conduction thresholds
   d. SRT of the test ear to the interaural attenuation

6. The need to mask during word-recognition testing is determined by comparing the
   a. hearing level of the test stimuli (PBHL) to the opposite ear bone-conduction thresholds
   b. SRT of the test ear to the interaural attenuation
   c. SRT of the test ear to the SRT of the nontest ear
   d. none of the above

7. Overmasking occurs during SRT testing when the
   a. test presentation level exceeds 95 dB
   b. interaural attenuation is greater than 60 dB
   c. test presentation level exceeds the SRT of the nontest ear
   d. effective masking level minus the patient's interaural attenuation equals or exceeds the bone-conduction thresholds of the test ear

8. Overmasking occurs during word-recognition testing when the
   a. test presentation level exceeds 95 dB
   b. interaural attenuation is greater than 60 dB
   c. test presentation level exceeds the SRT of the nontest ear
   d. effective masking level minus the patient's interaural attenuation meets or exceeds the bone-conduction thresholds of the test ear

9. The result of not masking, when required during speech-recognition threshold testing may be that the
   a. SRT was obtained by bone conduction in the nontest ear
   b. SRT was obtained by air conduction in the nontest ear
   c. SRT was actually lower (better) than what was observed
   d. none of the above

10. The result of not masking, when required during word-recognition testing may be that the
    a. word-recognition score is actually poorer than that which is observed
    b. nontest ear actually took the word-recognition test
    c. word-recognition test was actually taken by both ears
    d. all of the above

11. The result of overmasking during speech-recognition threshold testing may be that the
    a. SRT appears better than it truly is
    b. SRT appears worse than it truly is
    c. interaural attenuation is increased
    d. none of the above

12. The result of overmasking during word-recognition testing may be that the
    a. word-recognition score appears better than it truly is
    b. word-recognition score appears poorer than it truly is
    c. sensation level of the test is raised
    d. none of the above

13. When a patient's interaural attenuation is not known, it is safest to assume that it may be as little as _____ dB when testing with insert receivers
    a. 30
    b. 70
    c. 50
    d. 60

14. The air-bone gap of the masked ear must be added to minimum masking levels during speech-recognition testing because
    a. the conductive component of the loss attenuates the masking level
    b. the interaural attenuation is increased in conductive hearing losses
    c. masking is always needed when the test ear has a conductive hearing loss
    d. none of the above

15. Five decibels are often added to the usual sensation level for word recognition tests when masking is used to
    a. increase the interaural attenuation
    b. decrease the interaural attenuation
    c. account for cross-hearing
    d. offset central masking

16. If the interaural attenuation for speech can be determined to be greater than 40 dB when supra-aural earphones are used, it is better to use the larger number to
    a. increase the likelihood of undermasking
    b. decrease the likelihood of undermasking
    c. decrease the likelihood of overmasking
    d. increase the likelihood of overmasking

17. Overmasking during SRT testing results in the
    a. SRT of the nontest ear getting higher (poorer)
    b. SRT of the nontest ear getting lower (better)
    c. SRT of the test ear getting higher (poorer)
    d. SRT of the test ear getting lower (better)

18. One excellent means of minimizing the chances of undermasking or overmasking during speech audiometry is to
    a. test with insert receivers
    b. mask with insert receivers
    c. test and mask with insert receivers
    d. use supra-aural earphones

Answers—Unit B

Matching	*Outline*	*Multiple Choice*
1. h	**1.** G	**1.** b
2. d	**2.** F	**2.** d
3. l	**3.** A	**3.** b
4. a	**4.** D	**4.** a
5. n	**5.** C	**5.** c
6. f	**6.** E	**6.** a
7. b	**7.** B	**7.** d
8. i		**8.** d
9. o		**9.** a
10. g		**10.** d
11. m		**11.** b
12. k		**12.** b
13. c		**13.** b
14. e		**14.** a
15. j		**15.** d
		16. c
		17. c
		18. c

TABLE 5B.1   Chart for Masking

Test	Speech Right (Masking Left)		Test	Speech Left (Masking Right)	
	Masking needed?	*Min EM*		*Masking needed?*	*Min EM*
SRT-55 db	yes	45 dB	SRT-45 db	no	—
WRS-?%	yes	80 dB	WRS-?%	yes	75 dB

6 Electrophysiological Tests

Background

The word *immittance*, when applied to measurements at the tympanic membrane, is a combined form of the words *impedance* (the opposition to the flow of acoustic energy to the middle ear) and *admittance* (that acoustic energy passed by the tympanic membrane into the middle ear). It is a compromise in terminology. Three major tests can be carried out with modern electroacoustic immittance meters: (1) *static compliance*—a means of determining the degree of stiffness of the tympanic membrane and ossicular chain; (2) *tympanometry*—a measure of the compliance of the tympanic membrane with varying degrees of positive and negative pressure in the external auditory canal; (3) the *acoustic reflex threshold*—determination of the intensity of a sound required to contract the stapedius muscle when that sound is presented to the same ear as the probe, which senses tympanic membrane movement, or to the opposite ear. Acoustic reflexes can help in determining the site of pathology in sensorineural losses, approximation of degree of hearing loss in noncooperative patients, facial nerve integrity, and more.

The auditory brainstem response (ABR) currently is used not only as a test of hearing but also to help in determination of the site of auditory lesion. The development of averaging computers allows the presentation of numbers of stimuli so that the background activity can be averaged to near zero amplitude, while the series of wave peaks that signify responses at different points following stimulus introduction are increased in amplitude. All this serves to improve the signal-to-noise ratio. Responses are usually defined in terms of their latencies (time after stimulus onset), with the earliest responses occurring in the lower centers (e.g., the cochlea or brainstem) and the later responses in the auditory cortex.

The realization that it was possible to measure weak sounds in the external auditory canal that could be evoked by transient acoustic signals led to the rapid clinical implementation of transient-evoked auditory response audiometry. This procedure, which is maturing at a remarkable rate, has the promise to measure the hearing of newborn infants in a brief and economical fashion and to contribute to the diagnosis of the site of lesion within the auditory system.

Objectives

1. You should know and understand the terms in the matching exercise.
2. You should be able to fill in the outline, selecting items from the list provided.
3. You should understand the implications of static compliance, including its possible weaknesses as a measurement of true tympanic membrane function.
4. You should be able to interpret the different types of tympanograms, know how they are obtained, and what they imply.
5. You should know the implications of absent, elevated, and low sensation level acoustic reflex thresholds.
6. You should know some variations of the acoustic reflex test, including acoustic reflex decay, comparison of ipsilateral and contralateral acoustic reflex thresholds, and results of measurements made with different kinds of stimuli.
7. You should understand the different auditory evoked potential tests and what their latencies signify.
8. You should understand the principles of otoacoustic emissions and the tests available.
9. You should be able to answer the multiple-choice questions on electrophysiological measurements.

Matching

Match the term from the box on the right with its definition.

Definition

1. _____ The lowest intensity at which a stimulus produces an acoustic reflex

2. _____ The total contribution to impedance made by mass, stiffness, and frequency

3. _____ The VIIth cranial nerve, which runs from the brainstem to the stapedial tendon

4. _____ A small muscle whose insertion is in the neck of the stapes

5. _____ Measurement of the pressure-compliance function of the eardrum membrane

6. _____ Measurement of impedance or admittance of the eardrum membrane

7. _____ Contraction of the middle-ear muscles in response to sound

8. _____ A graph representing the pressure-compliance function of the eardrum membrane

9. _____ A small muscle whose insertion is in the neck of the malleus

10. _____ The inverse of stiffness

11. _____ That portion of impedance that is independent of frequency

12. _____ A unit of impedance measurement

13. _____ A decrease in the impedance of the eardrum membrane as a result of constant sound stimulation

14. _____ The ascending and descending pathways of the acoustic reflex

15. _____ Evoked potentials that appear 10 to 50 msec after signal onset (abbr.)

16. _____ Evoked potentials that appear 75 msec after signal onset with a large peak at a latency of 300 msec (abbr.)

Term

a. ABR
b. Acoustic reflex
c. Acoustic reflex arc
d. AMLR
e. ART
f. Auditory event-related
g. Compliance
h. ECochG
i. Facial nerve
j. Ground
k. Immittance
l. Latency-intensity
m. LER
n. Ohm
o. Reactance
p. Reference
q. Reflex decay
r. Resistance
s. Stapedius
t. Tensor tympani
u. Tympanogram
v. Tympanometry

Definition		*Term*
17. ____	The third electrode used in auditory evoked potential testing that prevents the body from acting as an antenna	**a.** ABR
		b. Acoustic reflex
		c. Acoustic reflex arc
18. ____	The electrode used in auditory evoked potential testing that is unaffected by electrical activity in the brain	**d.** AMLR
		e. ART
		f. Auditory event-related
		g. Compliance
19. ____	Evoked potentials that appear within the first 10 msec after signal onset (abbr.)	**h.** ECochG
		i. Facial nerve
		j. Ground
20. ____	Evoked potentials that occur almost immediately after signal onset	**k.** Immittance
		l. Latency-intensity
		m. LER
21. ____	A graph drawn as a function of the delay in appearance of wave V versus the intensity required to produce the wave	**n.** Ohm
		o. Reactance
		p. Reference
		q. Reflex decay
		r. Resistance
22. ____	Evoked potentials that appear about 100 msec after signal onset	**s.** Stapedius
		t. Tensor tympani
		u. Tympanogram
		v. Tympanometry

Outline

Electrophysiological Tests
Acoustic Immittance
Equipment
1. ____
2. ____
3. ____
4. ____
5. ____
6. ____
7. ____
8. ____
9. ____

Static Compliance
10. ____
11. ____
12. ____
13. ____

Tympanometry
14. ____
15. ____
16. ____
17. ____
18. ____

Acoustic Reflex
19. ____
20. ____
21. ____
22. ____

ABR
Stimulus
23. ____

Equipment
24. ____
25. ____

Response Latency
26. ____

ECochG
Stimulus
27. ____

Select From
A. Absent—bilateral conductive or severe sensorineural loss
B. Air pump
C. Averaging computer
D. Balance meter
E. Clicks or tone bursts
F. Compliance with TM "loose"
G. Compliance with TM "tight"
H. Contralateral earphone
I. Elevated—mild conductive loss
J. Low value—stiffness of TM and/or ossicular chain
K. Loudspeaker
L. Low SL—cochlear lesion
M. High value—interruption of ossicular chain, flaccid TM
N. Manometer
O. Microphone
P. Oscillator
Q. Potentiometer
R. Probe assembly
S. Promontory electrodes and amplifier
T. Pure tone
U. Reflex decay—retrocochlear lesion
V. Scalp electrodes and amplifier
W. Type A—normal ME
X. Type B—fluid in ME
Y. Type C—negative pressure in ME
Z. Type A_S—stiffness of ossicular chain
AA. Type A_D—very compliant TM
AB. 8 msec or less
AC. 10 msec or less
AD. 50–300 msec

ECochG
Equipment
28. ____
29. ____

Response Latency
30. ____

LER
Stimulus
31. ____

Equipment
32. ____
33. ____

Response Latency
34. ____

Select From

A. Absent—bilateral conductive or severe sensorineural loss
B. Air pump
C. Averaging computer
D. Balance meter
E. Clicks or tone bursts
F. Compliance with TM "loose"
G. Compliance with TM "tight"
H. Contralateral earphone
I. Elevated—mild conductive loss
J. Low value—stiffness of TM and/or ossicular chain
K. Loudspeaker
L. Low SL—cochlear lesion
M. High value—interruption of ossicular chain, flaccid TM
N. Manometer
O. Microphone
P. Oscillator
Q. Potentiometer
R. Probe assembly
S. Promontory electrodes and amplifier
T. Pure tone
U. Reflex decay—retrocochlear lesion
V. Scalp electrodes and amplifier
W. Type A—normal ME
X. Type B—fluid in ME
Y. Type C—negative pressure in ME
Z. Type A_S—stiffness of ossicular chain
AA. Type A_D—very compliant TM
AB. 8 msec or less
AC. 10 msec or less
AD. 50–300 msec

Activity

Sketch four different tympanograms on the following forms (Figures 6.1 to 6.4). Compare your graphs to the properly drawn tympanograms (Figures 6.5 to 6.8) at the end of this unit.

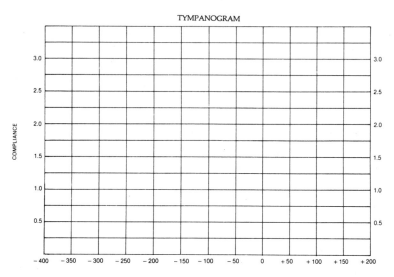

FIGURE 6.1

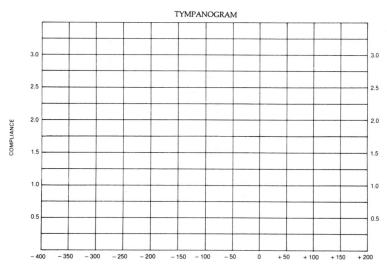

FIGURE 6.2

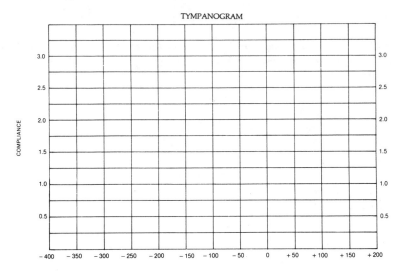

FIGURE 6.3

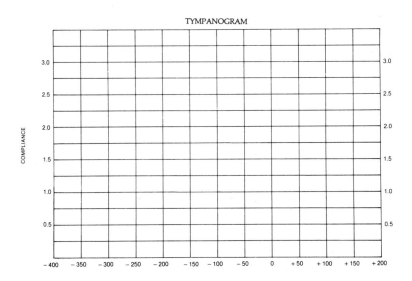

FIGURE 6.4

Multiple Choice

1. Theoretically, a patient with otosclerosis should show
   a. normal tympanic membrane compliance
   b. higher than normal tympanic membrane compliance
   c. lower than normal tympanic membrane compliance
   d. fluctuating tympanic membrane compliance
2. Absence of an acoustic reflex is probable in
   a. conductive hearing loss
   b. profound sensorineural hearing loss
   c. facial nerve paralysis
   d. all of the above
3. A patient has a 40 dB hearing loss caused by otosclerosis in the left ear. Acoustic reflexes with contralateral stimulation would probably show
   a. absent right, absent left
   b. present right, present left
   c. present right, absent left
   d. absent right, present left
4. Flat tympanograms may be attributed to any of the following except
   a. otitis media
   b. impacted cerumen
   c. interrupted ossicular chain
   d. probe opening against canal wall
5. A retracted tympanic membrane should yield a tympanogram type
   a. A
   b. B
   c. C
   d. D
6. Of the following, the most likely tympanogram to occur in the presence of otosclerosis is
   a. A_S
   b. A_D
   c. B
   d. C
7. A measured increase in compliance of the tympanic membrane may result from
   a. interrupted ossicular chain
   b. middle-ear infection
   c. perforated tympanic membrane
   d. cerumenosis
8. An acoustic reflex at a sensation level below 55 dB suggests
   a. no pathology
   b. middle-ear pathology
   c. cochlear pathology
   d. auditory nerve pathology

9. The portion of the ear responsible for the stiffness component of impedance in the plane of the tympanic membrane is the
   a. external ear
   b. ossicular ligaments
   c. ossicular mass
   d. fluid load on the stapes

10. Theoretically, an interrupted ossicular chain shows the tympanogram type
    a. A
    b. A_S
    c. A_D
    d. C

11. A tympanogram with maximum compliance at –200 daPa suggests
    a. normally aerated middle ear
    b. negative pressure in the middle ear
    c. positive pressure in the middle ear
    d. fluid in the middle ear

12. According to the impedance formula, early otosclerosis should result in an audio-metric configuration that is
    a. basically flat
    b. worse in the high frequencies
    c. worse in the mid-frequencies
    d. worse in the low frequencies

13. A tympanogram with no point of maximum compliance could result from
    a. fluid in the middle ear
    b. negative pressure in the middle ear
    c. a normally aerated middle ear
    d. positive pressure in the middle ear

14. In the use of an immittance meter with the probe in the right ear and the phone over the left ear, the contralateral acoustic reflex is designed to measure the
    a. Vth nerve left, reflex SL right
    b. recruitment right, decruitment left
    c. facial nerve left, reflex SL right
    d. facial nerve right, reflex SL left

15. Your patient has an intra-axial brainstem lesion on the right side but normal hearing for pure tones in both ears. Acoustic reflex results should be as follows:
    a. Contralateral: present left, absent right
       Ipsilateral: present left, absent right
    b. Contralateral: present right, present left
       Ipsilateral: absent right, present left
    c. Contralateral: absent right, absent left
       Ipsilateral: present right, present left
    d. Contralateral: present right, present left
       Ipsilateral: absent right, absent left

16. Acoustic reflexes at 5 dB SL suggest
    a. retrocochlear lesion
    b. cochlear lesion
    c. conductive lesion
    d. nonorganic hearing loss
17. The tympanic membrane is maximally compliant when
    a. middle-ear pressure equals outer-ear pressure
    b. middle-ear pressure is less than outer-ear pressure
    c. middle-ear pressure is greater than outer-ear pressure
    d. all of the above
18. Reflex decay to half amplitude at 500 Hz within 10 seconds suggests
    a. normal hearing
    b. conductive lesion
    c. cochlear lesion
    d. retrocochlear lesion
19. During measurements of static compliance, a patient's C_1 reading is 5.0 cc. This suggests
    a. interrupted ossicular chain
    b. otosclerosis
    c. tympanic membrane perforation
    d. otitis media
20. The component of impedance unrelated to frequency is
    a. resistance
    b. mass
    c. stiffness
    d. pi
21. Present in the contralateral acoustic reflex pathway but absent in the ipsilateral acoustic reflex pathway are the
    a. cochlear nuclei
    b. crossover pathways
    c. auditory nerves
    d. superior olivary complexes
22. Auditory brainstem response audiometry views responses to sounds that occur
    a. immediately after the stimulus
    b. 350 msec after the stimulus
    c. visually
    d. never
23. One very important device for performing auditory evoked response audiometry is a
    a. psychogalvanometer
    b. Wheatstone bridge
    c. averaging computer
    d. inductorium

24. During electrocochleography, the target electrode is not placed on the
a. round window
b. promontory
c. external auditory canal
d. mastoid process

25. During ABR the most reliable wave in normal-hearing adults is wave number
a. III
b. IV
c. V
d. VI

26. Middle latency responses are those that occur ____ msec after the presentation of the signal
a. 0–15
b. 15–50
c. 50–100
d. 100–300

27. The usual stimulus for ABR is a
a. click
b. pure tone
c. narrowband noise
d. wideband noise

28. During ABR the average electrical response is
a. 1–5 millivolts
b. 1–5 microvolts
c. 1–5 volts
d. none of the above

29. ECochG has an advantage over ABR in that
a. bone conduction can be done without masking
b. the test is less involved
c. the test takes less time
d. subjects need not be anesthetized

30. ABR results are an indication of
a. neural integrity
b. hearing loss in the 250 to 500 Hz range
c. hearing loss in the 6000 to 8000 Hz range
d. cortical function

31. The event-related potential is also called the
a. ABR
b. P300
c. AMLR
d. ECochG

32. Otoacoustic emissions occurring in the absence of external stimulation are called
a. SOAE
b. TEOAE
c. EOAE
d. DPOAE

33. Two primary tones are required when measuring
   a. SOAE
   b. TEOAE
   c. EOAE
   d. DPOAE
34. Otoacoustic emissions are usually absent in
   a. cochlear hearing loss
   b. conductive hearing loss
   c. VIIIth nerve hearing loss
   d. a & b
35. A patient with a moderate hearing loss and present evoked otoacoustic emissions probably has a(n)
   a. cochlear lesion
   b. conductive loss
   c. mixed loss
   d. VIIIth nerve loss
36. A patient with a mild-to-moderate sensorineural hearing loss with unexpectedly poor word-recognition scores, absence of all auditory brainstem responses, and normal otoacoustic emissions, probably has
   a. auditory neuropathy
   b. cochlear hearing loss
   c. acoustic neuroma
   d. conductive hearing loss

Answers

Matching	*Outline*	*Multiple Choice*
1. e	**1.** B	**1.** c
2. o	**2.** D	**2.** d
3. i	**3.** H	**3.** a
4. s	**4.** K	**4.** c
5. v	**5.** N	**5.** c
6. k	**6.** O	**6.** a
7. b	**7.** P	**7.** a
8. u	**8.** Q	**8.** c
9. t	**9.** R	**9.** b
10. g	**10.** J	**10.** c
11. v	**11.** M	**11.** b
12. n	**12.** G	**12.** d
13. q	**13.** F	**13.** a
14. c	**14.** W	**14.** d
15. d	**15.** X	**15.** c
16. f	**16.** Y	**16.** d
17. j	**17.** Z	**17.** a
18. p	**18.** AA	**18.** d
19. a	**19.** A	**19.** c
20. h	**20.** I	**20.** a
21. l	**21.** L	**21.** b
22. m	**22.** U	**22.** a
	23. E	**23.** c
	24. C	**24.** d
	25. V	**25.** c
	26. AC	**26.** b
	27. E	**27.** a
	28. C	**28.** b
	29. S	**29.** a
	30. AB	**30.** a
	31. T	**31.** b
	32. C	**32.** a
	33. V	**33.** d
	34. AD	**34.** d
		35. d
		36. a

Activity

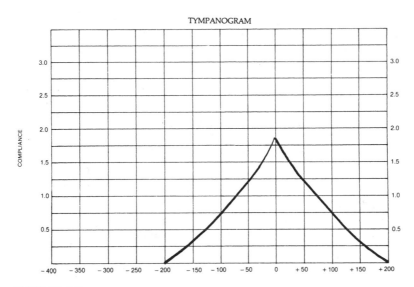

FIGURE 6.5

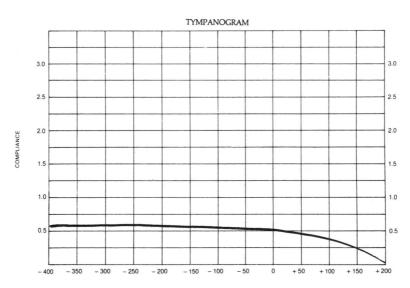

FIGURE 6.6

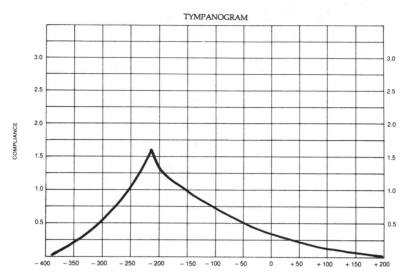

FIGURE 6.7

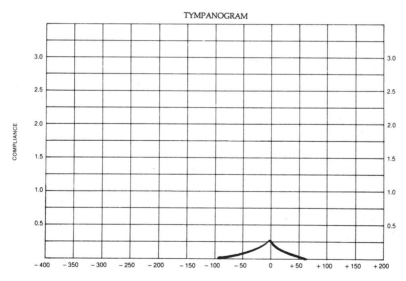

FIGURE 6.8

7 Behavioral Tests for Site of Lesion

Background

Through the years numbers of special tests have been developed based on different psychoacoustic phenomena. Lesions in various areas of the hearing system alter the responses on some of these tests. One phenomenon, loudness recruitment (the large increase in loudness with relatively small increases in intensity seen in patients with cochlear lesions), has led to the development of the Alternate Binaural Loudness Balance (ABLB) test. As an offshoot of the difference limen for intensity, the Short Increment Sensitivity Index (SISI) emerged as a means of determining cochlear lesions. This was later modified to test for retrocochlear sites. Studies examining the speed with which a continuous tone fades from audibility depending on auditory pathology resulted in a number of different tone-decay tests. By using the method of adjustment with the patient in control of the intensity of pure-tone signals, Békésy (automatic) audiometry has been used to track responses to auditory stimuli that may be different for continuous versus automatically pulsed tones. Although none of these tests is consistently accurate, when they are used together as a battery, the result is often a constellation that helps to identify the locus of disorder within the auditory system. Many of these tests are used less frequently today because of the introduction of electrophysiological procedures.

Objectives

1. You should know and understand the terms in the matching exercise.
2. You should be able to fill in the outline, selecting items from the list provided.
3. You should understand the principles underlying the ABLB test, the equipment required, and how the test is performed.
4. You should understand the principles underlying the SISI test, the equipment required, and how the test is performed.
5. You should understand the principles underlying the tone decay test, the equipment required, and how the test is performed.
6. You should understand the principles underlying Békésy audiometry, the equipment required, and how the test is performed.
7. You should be able to list the kinds of results on each of the above tests that theoretically would be expected from patients with normal hearing, as well as with conductive, cochlear, and retrocochlear lesions.
8. You should be able to complete the activities in this unit.
9. You should be able to answer the multiple-choice questions and understand the purposes and uses of behavioral tests for site of auditory lesion.

Matching

Match the term or abbreviation from the box on the right with its definition.

Definition

1. _____ A condition in which an intense sound is almost as loud to an impaired ear as it is to a normal ear

2. _____ A tone decay test carried out near the limits of an audiometer

3. _____ A test of perstimulatory adaptation

4. _____ Comparison of a comfortable level for pulsed and continuous tones, carried out on an automatic audiometer

5. _____ A test of loudness recruitment requiring the patient to have one normal and one hearing-impaired ear

6. _____ The less-than-normal growth of loudness of a signal as intensity is increased

7. _____ A plot for illustrating results on an ABLB or AMLB test

8. _____ A test to determine whether a patient can detect a change in the loudness of a tone when the intensity is increased by 1 dB

9. _____ A condition in which an intense sound is louder in an impaired ear than it is in a normal ear at the same intensity

10. _____ A procedure using automatic audiometry that compares a patient's thresholds for pulsed and continuous tones

11. _____ Perstimulatory adaptation to a pure tone

12. _____ The score (in percentage) on a test of word recognition

13. _____ The ability of a listener to barely detect small changes in intensity as changes in loudness

Term

a. ABLB
b. AMLB
c. BCL
d. Békésy audiometry
e. Decruitment
f. DLI
g. Hyperrecruitment
h. Laddergram
i. Partial recruitment
j. Recruitment
k. SISI
l. STAT
m. TDT
n. Tone decay
o. WRS

Definition

14. ____ A relatively large increase in loudness resulting from a small increase in intensity

15. ____ A test of loudness recruitment requiring the patient to have normal and impaired hearing at two frequencies in the same ear

Term

a. ABLB
b. AMLB
c. BCL
d. Békésy audiometry
e. Decruitment
f. DLI
g. Hyperrecruitment
h. Laddergram
i. Partial recruitment
j. Recruitment
k. SISI
l. STAT
m. TDT
n. Tone decay
o. WRS

Outline

Behavioral Tests

ABLB
Test for
1. ____

Type of Loss
2. ____

Results
3. ____
4. ____
5. ____
6. ____
7. ____

Equipment
8. ____

SISI
Test for
9. ____

Type of Loss
10. ____
11. ____

Results
12. ____
13. ____
14. ____

Equipment
15. ____

Tone Decay
Test for
16. ____
17. ____

Type of Loss
18. ____
19. ____

Results
20. ____
21. ____
22. ____

Select From

A. Audiometer and stopwatch
B. Békésy audiometer
C. Bilateral loss
D. Decruitment—retrocochlear
E. Detect 1 dB increments
F. Equal loudness in both ears at the same intensity
G. Hyperrecruitment—cochlear
H. No recruitment—conductive or retrocochlear
I. Partial recruitment—cochlear
J. Recruitment—cochlear
K. Separation of pulsed and continuous threshold tracings
L. SISI circuit
M. Tone fades to inaudibility
N. Tone loses musical quality
O. Type I—no decay—normal or conductive
P. Type II—slight decay—cochlear
Q. Type III—marked decay—retrocochlear
R. Two-channel audiometer
S. Unilateral loss
T. 0 to 25 percent—noncochlear
U. 30 to 70 percent—indeterminable
V. 75 to 100 percent—cochlear

Tone Decay
Equipment
23. ____

Békésy Audiometry
Test for
24. ____

Type of Loss
25. ____
26. ____

Equipment
27. ____

Select From

A. Audiometer and stopwatch
B. Békésy audiometer
C. Bilateral loss
D. Decruitment—retrocochlear
E. Detect 1 dB increments
F. Equal loudness in both ears at the same intensity
G. Hyperrecruitment—cochlear
H. No recruitment—conductive or retrocochlear
I. Partial recruitment—cochlear
J. Recruitment—cochlear
K. Separation of pulsed and continuous threshold tracings
L. SISI circuit
M. Tone fades to inaudibility
N. Tone loses musical quality
O. Type I—no decay—normal or conductive
P. Type II—slight decay—cochlear
Q. Type III—marked decay—retrocochlear
R. Two-channel audiometer
S. Unilateral loss
T. 0 to 25 percent—noncochlear
U. 30 to 70 percent—indeterminable
V. 75 to 100 percent—cochlear

Activities

ABLB

Six laddergrams are shown in Figure 7.1. The first is a model showing normal hearing in both ears. The other five show a 40 dB hearing loss in the right ear and normal hearing in the left ear. Show the theoretical levels in the left ear that are equal in loudness to 60 and 80 dB in the right ear for each of the following conditions: (B) no recruitment, (C) complete recruitment, (D) partial recruitment, (E) hyperrecruitment, and (F) decruitment. Compare your laddergrams to the correct ones (Figure 7.2) at the end of this unit.

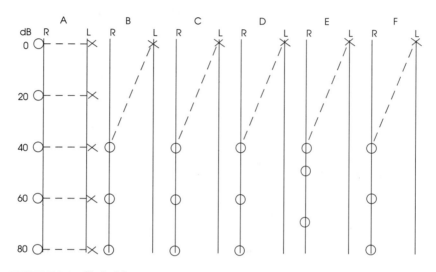

FIGURE 7.1   Six laddergrams.

Multiple Choice

1. A SISI score of 50 percent suggests
   a. cochlear lesion
   b. retrocochlear lesion
   c. conductive lesion
   d. unknown

2. When recruitment is present
   a. loudness grows so rapidly that a tone may be as loud in the impaired ear as it is in the normal ear at the same SPL
   b. loudness grows more slowly in the impaired ear than it does in a normal ear
   c. loudness grows more quickly than normal in the impaired ear but without complete recruitment
   d. there is no growth of loudness in the impaired ear

3. Normal-hearing individuals would be expected to get 100 percent SISI scores at _____ dB HL
   a. 10
   b. 20
   c. 40
   d. 80

4. The presence of loudness recruitment suggests
   a. conductive hearing loss
   b. normal hearing
   c. cochlear hearing loss
   d. retrocochlear loss

5. A patient has normal hearing in both ears but an VIIIth nerve lesion on the left side. SISI scores using 1 dB increments at 90 dB HL would probably be
   a. left 0 percent, right 0 percent
   b. left 100 percent, right 100 percent
   c. left 0 percent, right 100 percent
   d. left 100 percent, right 0 percent

6. In addition to threshold tracing, Békésy audiometry has been used diagnostically in tracking
   a. MCL
   b. WRS
   c. SRT
   d. 50 dB SL

7. Given a right cortical lesion, one would expect
   a. recruitment in the right ear
   b. recruitment in the left ear
   c. decruitment in the right ear
   d. decruitment in the left ear

8. During Békésy audiometry, a patient tracks the continuous tone at 50 dB HL and the interrupted tone at 70 dB HL. This would suggest
   a. conductive loss
   b. cochlear loss
   c. VIIIth nerve loss
   d. none of the above

9. Type II Békésy tracings are characterized by
   a. continuous poorer than pulsed at 1000 Hz and above
   b. continuous poorer than pulsed at 250 Hz and above
   c. continuous poorer than pulsed through the frequency range
   d. continuous and pulsed superimposed through the frequency range

10. The tone decay test that requires the patient to report a change in the quality of the tone is attributed to
    a. Green
    b. Olsen and Noffsinger
    c. Carhart
    d. Rosenberg

11. The tone decay test that is begun at 20 dB above the patient's threshold is attributed to
    a. Green
    b. Olsen and Noffsinger
    c. Carhart
    d. Rosenberg

12. The first tone decay test that could be completed in one minute per frequency is attributed to
    a. Green
    b. Olsen and Noffsinger
    c. Carhart
    d. Rosenberg

13. The high-intensity tone decay test is called
    a. STOP
    b. STAT
    c. START
    d. none of the above

14. In Békésy audiometry, separation between pulsed and continuous tracings is enhanced by
    a. sweeping from 100 to 10,000 Hz
    b. sweeping from 10,000 to 100 Hz
    c. using fixed frequency tracings
    d. not sweeping

15. To use the ABLB test the patient must have
    a. normal hearing in one ear and a hearing loss in the other ear
    b. normal hearing at one frequency in one ear and a hearing loss at a different frequency in the other ear
    c. normal hearing at one frequency and a hearing loss at a different frequency in the same ear
    d. hearing loss at all frequencies in both ears

16. The site-of-lesion test considered to have the greatest sensitivity is
   a. ABLB
   b. ABR
   c. SISI
   d. tone decay

Answers

Matching

1. i	**9.** g
2. l	**10.** d
3. m	**11.** n
4. c	**12.** o
5. a	**13.** f
6. e	**14.** j
7. h	**15.** b
8. k	

Outline

1. F	**15.** L
2. S	**16.** M
3. D	**17.** N
4. G	**18.** C
5. H	**19.** S
6. I	**20.** O
7. J	**21.** P
8. R	**22.** Q
9. E	**23.** A
10. C	**24.** K
11. S	**25.** C
12. T	**26.** S
13. U	**27.** B
14. V	

Mutiple Choice

1. d	**9.** a
2. a	**10.** a
3. d	**11.** b
4. c	**12.** d
5. c	**13.** b
6. a	**14.** b
7. d	**15.** a
8. d	**16.** b

Activity

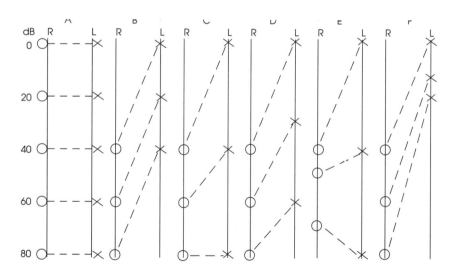

FIGURE 7.2

8 Hearing Tests for Children

Background

Although by age four or five years, many young children can take adult hearing tests that have been only slightly modified, others require special procedures and special equipment. There is no argument about whether hearing loss in children should be detected as early and accurately as possible. What is in debate are the means, methods, accuracy, and cost-effectiveness of different approaches. No hearing test on a noncooperative child is fool-proof, so a battery of procedures is best advised when diagnosis is critical.

Objectives

1. You should know and understand the terms in the matching exercise.
2. You should be able to fill in the outline, selecting items from the list provided.
3. You should know which hearing tests to use with children of different ages or different levels of function.
4. You should know what special equipment is necessary for specific tests.
5. You should be able to answer the multiple-choice questions on pediatric diagnosis.

Matching

Match the term from the box on the right with its definition.

Definition Term

1. _____ A set of criteria designed to help identify infants and young children at risk for hearing loss

2. _____ A system for checking the reliability of screening measures

3. _____ Observation of changes in the behavior of small children in response to sound

4. _____ A nonlinguistic speech audiometric measurement for assessing audibility of the acoustics of speech

5. _____ The use of tangible reinforcement to condition young children to take a hearing test

6. _____ Use of a light or picture to reinforce a child's response to sound

7. _____ The use of games or other play techniques in teaching children to respond during hearing tests

8. _____ A sound-field hearing test for children involving localization of the sound with visual reinforcement for head turning

9. _____ A form of conditioned audiometry using tangible reinforcers, such as food or tokens

10. _____ A startle response to sound in the form of an embracing movement

11. _____ Contraction of the muscles around the eyes in response to a loud sound

12. _____ The child's lowest response level (not necessarily the threshold) to an acoustic stimulus

Term

a. Auropalpebral reflex
b. Behavioral observation audiometry
c. Conditioned orientation reflex
d. High-risk registry
e. Ling six-sound test
f. Minimum response level
g. Moro reflex
h. Operant conditioning audiometry
i. Play audiometry
j. Tetrachoric table
k. TROCA
l. Visual reinforcement audiometry

Outline

Pediatric Diagnosis
Testing Infants

1. ____
2. ____
3. ____

Testing Infants and Small Children

4. ____
5. ____
6. ____
7. ____
8. ____

Testing Older Children (approximately 3 years and above)

9. ____
10. ____
11. ____
12. ____

Electrophysiological Tests (any age)

13. ____
14. ____
15. ____
16. ____

Select From

A. Auditory brainstem response
B. Auropalpebral reflex
C. Acoustic reflex threshold
D. Behavioral observation audiometry
E. Conditioned orientation reflex
F. High-risk registry
G. Moro reflex
H. Noisemakers
I. Operant conditioning audiometry
J. Otoacoustic emissions
K. Play audiometry
L. Speech-recognition threshold
M. Tympanometry
N. Visual response audiometry
O. Warblet
P. Word-recognition tests

Multiple Choice

1. The six sounds of the Ling six-sound test are
   a. f, s, j, r, v, and th
   b. oo (as in move), ee (as in beet), ah (as in father), sh, s, and m
   c. oo (as in book), i (as in kick), aa (as in back), f, th, and s
   d. f, s, sh, t, k, and r

2. Probably the easiest nonlanguage child to misdiagnose is the one with a hearing loss in
   a. the low frequencies
   b. the high frequencies
   c. the speech frequencies
   d. all frequencies

3. Difficulties encountered when using noisemakers to test neonates is control of
   a. distance
   b. intensity
   c. frequency
   d. all of the above

4. The "eye blink response" from infants to loud sounds is called
   a. ABR
   b. COR
   c. Moro reflex
   d. APR

5. Minimum sensory deprivation syndrome may be suspected of children with
   a. repeated otitis media
   b. Rh incompatibility
   c. family history of hearing loss
   d. prematurity

6. Present neonatal screening protocol recommends that it should be performed
   a. on all neonates
   b. on neonates failing one part of the high-risk registry
   c. on neonates who seem not to hear
   d. on no neonates

7. Electrodermal audiometry has been largely abandoned as a test for small children because
   a. the stimuli are too noxious for most children
   b. results were often unreliable
   c. further habilitation efforts are often affected adversely because of the child's fears
   d. all of the above

8. COR utilizes
   a. one loudspeaker and one lighted doll
   b. one loudspeaker and two lighted dolls
   c. two loudspeakers and one lighted doll
   d. two loudspeakers and two lighted dolls

9. ABR has some limits in pediatric diagnosis because
   a. it does not provide information about hearing in the low frequencies
   b. it does not provide information about hearing in the high frequencies
   c. it provides information only about the speech frequencies
   d. none of the above

10. Normal speech-detection thresholds in children do not necessarily mean normal hearing because
    a. hearing may be normal only in the low- or high-frequency range
    b. the SRT may be poorer than the SDT
    c. both a and b
    d. none of the above

11. An infant's startle response to a loud sound may mean
    a. normal hearing in both ears
    b. normal hearing in one ear
    c. a moderate hearing loss with recruitment
    d. all of the above

12. Ideally, public school hearing screening programs would include
    a. pure-tone screening
    b. pure-tone screening and tympanometry
    c. pure-tone screening, tympanometry, and acoustic reflexes
    d. pure-tone screening, tympanometry, acoustic reflexes, and SRTs

13. In operant conditioning the reinforcer should
    a. immediately follow the response
    b. be tangible
    c. be positive
    d. all of the above

14. Otoacoustic emissions have an advantage in neonatal hearing testing in that they
    a. are stable and reliable
    b. can be measured when the child is asleep or awake
    c. are unaffected by medications used to put a child to sleep
    d. all the above

Answers

Matching
1. d
2. j
3. b
4. e
5. h
6. l
7. i
8. c
9. k
10. g
11. a
12. f

Outline
1. B
2. F
3. O
4. D
5. G
6. H
7. E
8. N
9. I
10. K
11. L
12. P
13. A
14. C
15. J
16. M

Multiple Choice
1. b
2. b
3. d
4. d
5. a
6. a
7. d
8. d
9. a
10. a
11. d
12. c
13. d
14. d

9

The Outer Ear

Background

The outer ear is the most visible part of the auditory system and is made up primarily of a funnel-like appendage, a resonating tube, and a vibrating membrane. Its function is to gather sound waves from the environment and allow them to propagate to the eardrum membrane. Any obstruction that blocks the passageway can cause a conductive hearing loss.

Objectives

1. You should know and understand the terms in the matching exercise.
2. You should be able to fill in the outline, selecting items from the list provided.
3. You should be able to label parts of the outer ear and tympanic membrane in Figures 9.1, 9.2, and 9.3.
4. You should be able to answer the multiple-choice questions and understand the anatomy and physiology of the outer ear, as well as the causes of disorders that produce conductive hearing loss.

Matching

Match the term from the box on the right with its definition.

Definition

1. _____ Earwax
2. _____ A special light designed for looking into the ear
3. _____ Absence of the pinna
4. _____ The same as pars flaccida
5. _____ Inflammation of the external ear
6. _____ The tense portion of the tympanic membrane, making up its largest area and consisting of three layers
7. _____ The appendage of the external ear consisting of cartilage
8. _____ Surgery to repair the tympanic membrane
9. _____ The point of the tympanic membrane that is approximately in the center
10. _____ Closure of a body orifice that is normally open
11. _____ The flabby portion of the tympanic membrane found near the top
12. _____ The membrane that vibrates to allow sound to enter the middle ear from the outer ear
13. _____ Ear pain
14. _____ The channel that conducts sound from the auricle to the tympanic membrane
15. _____ Failure of a portion of the anatomy to develop

Term

a. Agenesis
b. Anotia
c. Atresia
d. Auricle
e. Cerumen
f. External auditory canal
g. External otitis
h. Myringoplasty
i. Otalgia
j. Otoscope
k. Pars flaccida
l. Pars tensa
m. Shrapnell's membrane
n. Tympanic membrane
o. Umbo

Outline

The Outer Ear
Anatomy

1. _____
2. _____
3. _____
4. _____

Disorders

5. _____
6. _____
7. _____
8. _____
9. _____
10. _____

Surgical Treatment

11. _____
12. _____

Select From

A. Atresia
B. Bony external ear canal
C. Cartilaginous external ear canal
D. Foreign bodies
E. Infections
F. Myringoplasty
G. Perforations
H. Pinna
I. Tympanic membrane
J. Tympanoplasty
K. Tumors
L. Wax

Activities

Label the parts of the pinna, outer ear, and tympanic membrane in the figures that follow. Select the terms from the lists provided.

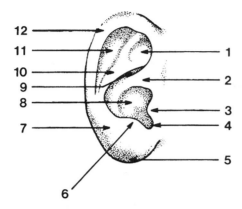

FIGURE 9.1. The pinna (auricle).

Label		*Term*
1. _____		**A.** Antihelix
2. _____		**B.** Antitragus
3. _____		**C.** Cavum concha
4. _____		**D.** Crus of helix
5. _____		**E.** Cymba concha
6. _____		**F.** Helix
7. _____		**G.** Intertragal notch
8. _____		**H.** Lobe
9. _____		**I.** Scaphoid fossa
10. _____		**J.** Tragus
11. _____		**K.** Triangular fossa
12. _____		

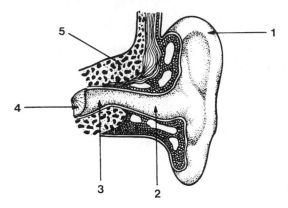

FIGURE 9.2.   The outer ear.

Label	*Term*
1. _____	**A.** Auricle (pinna)
2. _____	**B.** Bony external auditory canal
3. _____	**C.** Cartilaginous external auditory canal
4. _____	**D.** Mastoid air cells
5. _____	**E.** Tympanic membrane

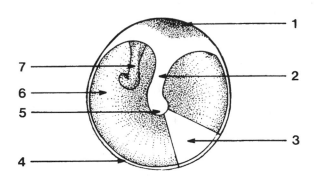

FIGURE 9.3.   The tympanic membrane.

Label	*Term*
1. _____	**A.** Annular ligament
2. _____	**B.** Cone of light
3. _____	**C.** Long process of incus
4. _____	**D.** Manubrium of malleus
5. _____	**E.** Pars flaccida
6. _____	**F.** Pars tensa
7. _____	**G.** Umbo

Multiple Choice

1. Cerumen is produced in the
   a. entire external auditory canal
   b. cartilaginous external auditory canal
   c. osseous external auditory canal
   d. temporomandibular joint
2. Congenital absence of the external auditory canal is called
   a. microtia
   b. stenosis
   c. minutia
   d. atresia
3. The portion of the tympanic membrane in which the malleus is embedded is the
   a. umbo
   b. annulus
   c. cone of light
   d. pars tensa
4. A large central perforation of the tympanic membrane theoretically results in hearing that is
   a. normal
   b. slightly to moderately impaired
   c. severely impaired
   d. profoundly impaired
5. A term for a bacterial infection of the outer ear is
   a. otomycosis
   b. cerumen in the lumen
   c. otitis media
   d. external otitis
6. The portion of the tympanic membrane that does not contain the fibrocartilaginous layer is the
   a. umbo
   b. pars tensa
   c. pars flaccida
   d. annulus
7. In air-conduction audiometry, a loss of the pinna results in
   a. no measurable hearing loss
   b. mild sensorineural hearing loss
   c. mild conductive hearing loss
   d. mild mixed hearing loss
8. The point of maximum retraction of the tympanic membrane is the
   a. annulus
   b. concha
   c. umbo
   d. pars flaccida

9. The resonant frequency of the external auditory canal is
   a. 500–2000 Hz
   b. 3000–5000 Hz
   c. 8000–10,000 Hz
   d. 10,000–12,000 Hz

10. The innermost layer of the tympanic membrane (on the middle-ear side) is covered with
    a. epidermis
    b. fibrous material
    c. mucous membrane
    d. muscle

11. The cone of light of the tympanic membrane is
    a. superior-anterior
    b. superior-posterior
    c. inferior-anterior
    d. inferior-posterior

12. Narrowing of the external auditory canal is called
    a. atresia
    b. stenosis
    c. otitis
    d. otomycosis

Answers

Matching
1. e
2. j
3. b
4. m
5. g
6. l
7. d
8. h
9. o
10. c
11. k
12. n
13. i
14. f
15. a

Outline
1. B
2. C
3. H
4. I
5. A
6. D
7. E
8. G
9. K
10. L
11. F
12. J

Multiple Choice
1. b
2. d
3. d
4. b
5. d
6. c
7. a
8. c
9. b
10. c
11. c
12. b

Activities

Pinna
1. K
2. D
3. J
4. G
5. H
6. B
7. F
8. C
9. E
10. A
11. I
12. F

Outer Ear
1. A
2. C
3. B
4. E
5. D

Tympanic Membrane
1. E
2. D
3. B
4. A
5. G
6. F
7. C

10 The Middle Ear

Background

The middle ear is a tiny air-filled space whose function is to match the impedance of air in the outer ear canal to fluid in the inner ear. Because the middle ear is in the conductive portion of the auditory system, abnormalities in this region affect a patient's air-conduction threshold with minimal effects on bone conduction. When only the middle ear is involved, a hearing loss should be purely conductive and may range from very mild to moderately severe. Air-bone gaps greater than 60 dB are quite rare. If both the middle ear and inner ear are disordered, either from common or unrelated causes, a mixed hearing loss may be present. Damage to the middle ear and other portions of the auditory system are not mutually exclusive. Dysfunction of the middle ear may result from disease, trauma, or hereditary conditions.

Objectives

1. You should know and understand the terms in the matching exercise.
2. You should be able to fill in the outline, selecting items from the list provided.
3. You should be able to label the different parts of the middle ear shown in Figure 10.1.
4. You should be able to answer the multiple-choice questions and understand the anatomy and physiology of the middle ear as well as the causes of disorders that produce conductive hearing loss.

Matching

Match the term from the box on the right with its definition.

Definition

1. _____ The largest of the ossicles, which is attached to the tympanic membrane

2. _____ An operation to reverse hearing loss caused by otosclerosis, carried out by breaking the stapes footplate free

3. _____ An artifact in bone conduction in patients with otosclerosis

4. _____ A surgical procedure to restore middle-ear function

5. _____ The VIIth cranial nerve

6. _____ The second bone in the ossicular chain that connects the malleus to the stapes

7. _____ The chain of three tiny bones in the middle ear

8. _____ Sterile fluid accumulation in the middle ear

9. _____ An operation to remove infection from the mastoid

10. _____ A space in the superior portion of the middle ear

11. _____ The Vth cranial nerve

12. _____ A small muscle that can impede movement of the malleus

13. _____ Inflammation of the mastoid

14. _____ An operation designed to improve hearing loss caused by otosclerosis by removing the stapes and replacing it with a prosthesis

15. _____ The attic of the middle-ear space

16. _____ The moist lining of the middle-ear space

17. _____ Infection of the middle ear

18. _____ In anatomy, a leg, as of the stapes

19. _____ Formation of spongy bone that may affect the normal movement of the stapes

Term

a. Aditus
b. Carhart notch
c. Cholesteatoma
d. Crus
e. Epitympanic recess
f. Eustachian tube
g. Facial nerve
h. Fenestration
i. Incus
j. Malleus
k. Mastoidectomy
l. Mastoiditis
m. Mucous membrane
n. Myringotomy
o. Ossicles
p. Otitis media
q. Otosclerosis
r. Oval window
s. Round window
t. Serous effusion
u. Stapedectomy
v. Stapedius muscle
w. Stapes
x. Stapes mobilization
y. Tensor tympani muscle
z. Trigeminal nerve
aa. Tympanoplasty
ab. Tympanosclerosis

Definition

20. _____ Incision into the tympanic membrane, usually to remove fluid

21. _____ A membrane separating the middle ear from the inner ear

22. _____ A channel connecting the middle ear to the nasopharynx

23. _____ Calcium formations between layers of the tympanic membrane or in the middle ear, often caused by infection

24. _____ The smallest of the ossicles, which stands in the oval window

25. _____ An older operation to correct hearing loss from otosclerosis

26. _____ A membrane, supporting the footplate of the stapes, that separates the middle ear from the inner ear

27. _____ A small muscle, connected to the stapes, that impedes movement of the ossicles when it is contracted

28. _____ A collection of fats and other debris in the middle ear, usually caused by infection

Term

a. Aditus
b. Carhart notch
c. Cholesteatoma
d. Crus
e. Epitympanic recess
f. Eustachian tube
g. Facial nerve
h. Fenestration
i. Incus
j. Malleus
k. Mastoidectomy
l. Mastoiditis
m. Mucous membrane
n. Myringotomy
o. Ossicles
p. Otitis media
q. Otosclerosis
r. Oval window
s. Round window
t. Serous effusion
u. Stapedectomy
v. Stapedius muscle
w. Stapes
x. Stapes mobilization
y. Tensor tympani muscle
z. Trigeminal nerve
aa. Tympanoplasty
ab. Tympanosclerosis

Outline

The Middle Ear
Anatomy
1. ____
2. ____
3. ____
4. ____
5. ____
6. ____
7. ____

Bones
8. ____
9. ____
10. ____

Muscles
11. ____
12. ____

Disorders
13. ____
14. ____
15. ____
16. ____
17. ____
18. ____

Surgical Treatment
19. ____
20. ____
21. ____
22. ____
23. ____
24. ____

Select From
A. Aditus ad antrum
B. Congenital abnormalities
C. Epitympanic recess
D. Eustachian tube
E. Fenestration
F. Fractures
G. Incus
H. Malleus
I. Mastoidectomy
J. Middle-ear space
K. Myringotomy
L. Otitis media
M. Otosclerosis
N. Oval window
O. Round window
P. Serous effusion
Q. Stapedectomy
R. Stapes
S. Stapes mobilization
T. Stapedius
U. Tensor tympani
V. Tympanic membrane
W. Tympanoplasty
X. Tympanosclerosis

Activity

Select the terms from the list provided and label the parts of the middle ear in Figure 10.1.

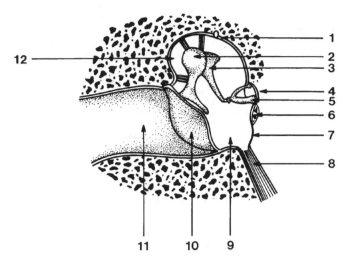

FIGURE 10.1.   The middle ear.

Label		*Term*
1. _____		**A.** Aditus ad antrum
2. _____		**B.** Epitympanic recess
3. _____		**C.** Eustachian tube
4. _____		**D.** External auditory canal
5. _____		**E.** Incus
6. _____		**F.** Malleus
7. _____		**G.** Middle-ear space
8. _____		**H.** Oval window
9. _____		**I.** Promontory
10. _____		**J.** Round window
11. _____		**K.** Stapes
12. _____		**L.** Tympanic membrane

Multiple Choice

1. The chain of bones in the middle ear is called the
   a. malleus
   b. incus
   c. stapes
   d. ossicles

2. Stapedectomy and stapedotomy have replaced stapes mobilization because
   a. there is less possibility of refixation
   b. the potential air-bone gap is small
   c. the operation is tolerated better
   d. it is less dangerous to perform

3. The general classification of surgical procedures for repairing damage of middle ear structures is
   a. tympanoplasty
   b. stapedialplasty
   c. rhinoplasty
   d. otoplasty

4. A pseudotumor in the middle ear composed of skin and fatty tissue is called
   a. otitis externa
   b. otosclerosis
   c. otitis media
   d. cholesteatoma

5. Which of the following is *not* a usual treatment for serous effusion?
   a. pressure-equalizing tubes
   b. mastoidectomy
   c. myringotomy
   d. decongestant medication

6. Pressure-equalizing tubes are designed to function primarily as an artificial
   a. ear canal
   b. mastoid
   c. eustachian tube
   d. middle ear

7. The most popular surgical treatment for otosclerosis is
   a. fenestration
   b. tympanoplasty
   c. stapedotomy
   d. stapes mobilization

8. The manubrium is part of the
   a. malleus
   b. incus
   c. stapes
   d. eustachian tube

9. The eustachian tube connects the middle ear with the
   a. outer ear
   b. inner ear
   c. nasopharynx
   d. nose
10. Nonbacterial otitis media usually results from
    a. a blocked eustachian tube
    b. nasopharyngitis
    c. otitis media
    d. otosclerosis
11. Otosclerosis is
    a. equally common in men and women
    b. most common in men
    c. most common in women
    d. most common in children
12. Fluid in the middle-ear space may result from
    a. a blocked eustachian tube
    b. infection entering the middle ear via the eustachian tube
    c. infection entering the middle ear via the bloodstream
    d. all of the above
13. Hearing speech better in a noisy place than in a quiet place is a symptom of
    a. normal hearing
    b. conductive hearing loss
    c. sensorineural hearing loss
    d. none of the above
14. The Carhart notch is usually associated with
    a. otosclerosis
    b. bacterial otitis media
    c. serous effusion
    d. a blocked eustachian tube
15. Given a moderate conductive hearing loss in the right ear and normal hearing in the left ear, otoacoustic emissions are expected to be
    a. absent in both ear
    b. present in both ears
    c. present in the right ear, absent in the left ear
    d. present in the left ear, absent in the right ear

Answers

Matching	*Outline*	*Activity*	*Multiple Choice*
1. j	**1.** A	**1.** A	**1.** d
2. x	**2.** C	**2.** F	**2.** a
3. b	**3.** D	**3.** E	**3.** a
4. aa	**4.** J	**4.** H	**4.** d
5. g	**5.** N	**5.** K	**5.** b
6. i	**6.** O	**6.** I	**6.** c
7. o	**7.** V	**7.** J	**7.** c
8. t	**8.** G	**8.** C	**8.** a
9. k	**9.** H	**9.** G	**9.** c
10. e	**10.** R	**10.** L	**10.** a
11. z	**11.** T	**11.** D	**11.** c
12. y	**12.** U	**12.** B	**12.** d
13. l	**13.** B		**13.** b
14. u	**14.** F		**14.** a
15. a	**15.** L		**15.** d
16. m	**16.** M		
17. p	**17.** P		
18. d	**18.** X		
19. q	**19.** E		
20. n	**20.** I		
21. s	**21.** K		
22. f	**22.** Q		
23. ab	**23.** S		
24. w	**24.** W		
25. h			
26. r			
27. v			
28. c			

CHAPTER

11 The Inner Ear

UNIT A: STRUCTURE, FUNCTION, AND DISORDERS

Background

The inner ear is often called a *labyrinth*, which is Greek for a series of winding passages. Although extremely tiny, it is a myriad of hydromechanical and neuroelectrical activities. Through its vestibular apparatus the inner ear provides the brain with the sensation of the head's position and motion in space. Through the cochlea the inner ear converts the mechanical acoustical vibrations of the middle ear into a form of energy, which the brain ultimately perceives as sound. Damage to the cochlea causes hearing losses that are termed sensorineural. Cochlear hearing losses result from a wide variety of causes and can occur at any age.

Objectives

1. You should know and understand the terms in the matching exercise.
2. You should be able to fill in the outline, selecting items from the list provided.
3. You should be able to label the different parts of the inner ear as shown in Figures 11A.1 and 11A.2.
4. You should be able to answer the multiple-choice questions and understand the anatomy and physiology of the inner ear as well as the causes of disorders that produce sensorineural hearing loss in the inner ear.

Matching

Match the term from the box on the right with its definition.

Definition

1. _____ The efferent portion of a neuron

2. _____ A procedure designed to monitor spontaneous or induced nystagmus

3. _____ Fluid contained in the vestibular and cochlear portions of the bony labyrinth that surrounds the membranous labyrinth

4. _____ The central portion of a nerve cell

5. _____ A vascular strip along the outer wall of the scala media that supplies oxygen to the cochlea

6. _____ The cavity of the inner ear that contains the organs of equilibrium

7. _____ Nerves that carry impulses from the periphery to the brain

8. _____ Three loops within the vestibule that monitor angular acceleration

9. _____ The smaller of two sacs in the vestibule that is responsible for sensing linear acceleration

10. _____ The cochlear duct containing the organ of Corti

11. _____ The widened ends of the semicircular canals that contain the cristae

12. _____ Oscillatory movement of the eyes

13. _____ Fluid contained in the membranous labyrinth

14. _____ The membrane separating the scala media from the scala tympani and supporting the organ of Corti

15. _____ The interconnecting canals in the temporal bone that contain perilymph in which is found the membranous labyrinth

16. _____ The branching portion of a neuron that carries impulses to the cell body

Term

a. Afferent
b. Ampulla
c. Axon
d. Basilar membrane
e. Cell body
f. Cochlea
g. Dendrite
h. Efferent
i. Electronystagmography
j. Endolymph
k. Helicotrema
l. Labyrinth
m. Neuron
n. Nystagmus
o. Perilymph
p. Reissner's membrane
q. Saccule
r. Scala media
s. Scala tympani
t. Scala vestibuli
u. Semicircular canals
v. Stria vascularis
w. Tectorial membrane
x. Utricle
y. Vertigo
z. Vestibule

Definition

17. _____ The duct in the inner ear above the scala media that contains perilymph

18. _____ The larger of two sacs in the vestibule that is responsible for sensing linear acceleration

19. _____ Nerves that carry impulses from the brain to the periphery

20. _____ The sensation of true turning or spinning

21. _____ The membrane separating the scala vestibuli from the scala media

22. _____ The membrane in the scala media above the organ of Corti into which the tips of the hair cells are embedded

23. _____ The duct below the scala media that is filled with perilymph

24. _____ An opening at the apical end of the cochlea connecting the scala vestibuli with the scala tympani

25. _____ A cell specialized for conveying nerve impulses

26. _____ A cavity in the temporal bone containing the end organ of hearing

Term

a. Afferent
b. Ampulla
c. Axon
d. Basilar membrane
e. Cell body
f. Cochlea
g. Dendrite
h. Efferent
i. Electronystagmography
j. Endolymph
k. Helicotrema
l. Labyrinth
m. Neuron
n. Nystagmus
o. Perilymph
p. Reissner's membrane
q. Saccule
r. Scala media
s. Scala tympani
t. Scala vestibuli
u. Semicircular canals
v. Stria vascularis
w. Tectorial membrane
x. Utricle
y. Vertigo
z. Vestibule

Outline

The Inner Ear
Anatomy of the Cochlea

1. ____
2. ____
3. ____
4. ____
5. ____
6. ____
7. ____
8. ____
9. ____
10. ____
11. ____
12. ____
13. ____

Anatomy of the Vestibule

14. ____
15. ____
16. ____
17. ____
18. ____
19. ____

Disorders

20. ____
21. ____
22. ____
23. ____
24. ____
25. ____
26. ____
27. ____
28. ____

Select from

A. Ampulla
B. Anoxia
C. Basilar membrane
D. Cortilymph
E. Crista
F. Drug-induced
G. Ductus reuniens
H. Hair cells
I. Helictorema
J. Macula
K. Méniére disease
L. Noise-induced
M. Organ of Corti
N. Otosclerosis
O. Prenatal viral infections
P. Presbycusis
Q. Postnatal viral infections
R. Reissner's membrane
S. Saccule
T. Scala media
U. Scala tympani
V. Scala vestibuli
W. Semicircular canals
X. Skull fracture
Y. Spiral ligament
Z. Stria vascularis
AA. Tectorial membrane
AB. Utricle

Activities

Label the parts of the labyrinth and cross section of the cochlea in the figures that follow. Select the names from the lists provided.

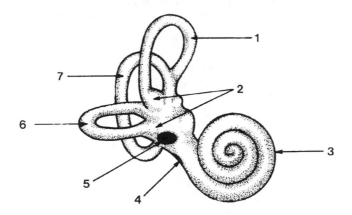

FIGURE 11A.1.   The labyrinth.

Label		*Term*
1. _____		**A.** Ampullae
2. _____		**B.** Cochlea
3. _____		**C.** Horizontal (lateral) semicircular canal
4. _____		**D.** Inferior (posterior) semicircular canal
5. _____		**E.** Oval window
6. _____		**F.** Round window
7. _____		**G.** Superior (anterior) semicircular canal

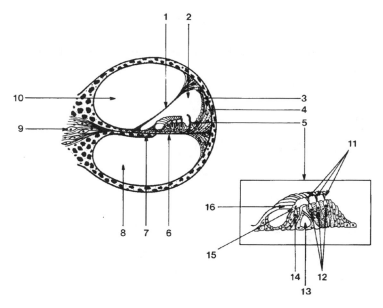

FIGURE 11A.2. **Cross section of the cochlea.**

Label	Term
1. _____	**A.** Basilar membrane
2. _____	**B.** Inner hair cell cilia
3. _____	**C.** Inner hair cells
4. _____	**D.** Organ of Corti
5. _____	**E.** Outer hair cell cilia
6. _____	**F.** Outer hair cells
7. _____	**G.** Reissner's membrane
8. _____	**H.** Scala media (endolymph)
9. _____	**I.** Scala tympani (perilymph)
10. _____	**J.** Scala vestibuli (perilymph)
11. _____	**K.** Spiral ganglion
12. _____	**L.** Spiral lamina
13. _____	**M.** Spiral ligament
14. _____	**N.** Stria vascularis
15. _____	**O.** Tectorial membrane
16. _____	**P.** Tunnel of Corti

Multiple Choice

1. A device used to measure oscillatory movement of the eyes in response to caloric stimulation is called an
   a. electronystagmograph
   b. electroencephalograph
   c. electromyograph
   d. audiograph

2. The stria vascularis does not
   a. carry blood
   b. support hair cells
   c. produce a DC potential
   d. produce endolymph

3. The type of cerebral palsy most associated with sensorineural hearing loss is
   a. spasticity
   b. rigidity
   c. athetosis
   d. ataxia

4. Angular acceleration is measured in
   a. cm/sec^2
   b. cm/sec
   c. degrees/sec
   d. degrees/sec^2

5. The macula is the end organ located within the
   a. semicircular canals
   b. cochlea
   c. utricle
   d. brain

6. ____ does not make up a wall of the cochlear duct
   a. bony shelf
   b. tectorial membrane
   c. basilar membrane
   d. Reissner's membrane

7. Endolymph is found in the
   a. tectorial membrane
   b. scala vestibuli
   c. scala media
   d. scala tympani

8. The fluid surrounding the membranous labyrinth is called
   a. cortilymph
   b. perilymph
   c. endolymph
   d. lymph

9. The portion of the inner ear that responds to angular acceleration is called
   a. macula
   b. semicircular canals
   c. organ of Corti
   d. utricle
10. The central core around which the cochlea winds is the
    a. modiolus
    b. Reissner's membrane
    c. helicotrema
    d. basilar membrane
11. The tips of the outer hair cells are embedded in
    a. Reissner's membrane
    b. the bony shelf
    c. the tectorial membrane
    d. the basilar membrane
12. The most common postnatal cause of bilateral hearing loss from viral infection is
    a. rubeola (measles)
    b. rubella (German measles)
    c. pertussis (whooping cough)
    d. varicella (chicken pox)
13. Linear acceleration is measured in
    a. cm/sec^2
    b. cm/sec
    c. degrees/sec
    d. degrees/sec^2
14. Which of the following is not considered a perinatal cause of hearing loss?
    a. anoxia
    b. trauma
    c. rubella
    d. prolonged labor
15. Deprivation of oxygen, which may cause damage to the cochlea (and the brain), is called
    a. dysphemia
    b. dyscalculia
    c. dyslogia
    d. anoxia
16. The small opening allowing passage of perilymph from scala vestibuli to scala tympani is called
    a. modiolus
    b. stria vascularis
    c. spiral ligament
    d. helicotrema
17. The number of turns of the cochlea is
    a. 2
    b. 2½
    c. 3
    d. 3½

18. The structure just medial to the oval window is the
    a. cochlea
    b. semicircular canals
    c. vestibule
    d. helix
19. The crista is the end organ of the
    a. utricle
    b. saccule
    c. cochlea
    d. semicircular canals
20. Rapid back and forth movement of the eyes is called
    a. vertigo
    b. nystagmus
    c. dizziness
    d. near sightedness
21. The fluid contained in the membranous labyrinth is
    a. perilymph
    b. cortilymph
    c. blood
    d. endolymph
22. The end organ of hearing is the
    a. crista
    b. macula
    c. helicotrema
    d. organ of Corti
23. The portion of the inner ear responsible for linear acceleration is the
    a. semicircular canals
    b. utricle and saccule
    c. crista
    d. organ of Corti
24. During caloric testing when a normal left ear is stimulated with cold water, the eye beat is
    a. right
    b. left
    c. random
    d. unpredictable
25. Endolymph differs from perilymph because in endolymph
    a. potassium concentration is greater
    b. potassium concentration is less
    c. sodium concentration is greater
    d. resting microvoltage is less
26. Screening for hearing loss in the ultra-high-frequency range is often useful in detecting hearing loss caused by
    a. noise
    b. infection
    c. Méniére disease
    d. ototoxic drugs

27. Méniére disease is associated with
    a. bilateral hearing loss, good speech recognition
    b. unilateral hearing loss, poor speech recognition
    c. unilateral hearing loss, good speech recognition
    d. normal vestibular findings
28. Hereditary cochlear hearing loss resulting from genetic and environmental interactions is called
    a. homozygous
    b. hereditodegenerative
    c. multifactorial
    d. x-linked
29. Rh interactions put a baby at risk when
    a. mother is positive, father is positive
    b. mother is negative, father is negative
    c. mother is positive, father is negative
    d. mother is negative, father is positive
30. Presbycusis is hearing loss associated with
    a. aging
    b. noise
    c. bacterial infection
    d. viral infection
31. Sudden unilateral cochlear hearing loss may be caused by
    a. spasm of the internal auditory artery
    b. Méniére disease
    c. labyrinthitis
    d. all of the above
32. A hearing loss due to aging that is associated with loss of outer hair cells and supporting cells in the basal turn of the cochlea is called
    a. sensory presbycusis
    b. neural presbycusis
    c. strial presbycusis
    d. cochlear conductive presbycusis
33. Associated with cochlear hearing loss is
    a. loudness decruitment
    b. negative SISI scores
    c. loudness recruitment
    d. rapid tone decay
34. The ABR latency-intensity function for wave V expected in cochlear hearing losses is
    a. increased, primarily at high intensities
    b. increased, primarily at low intensities
    c. decreased, primarily at high intensities
    d. decreased, primarily at low intensities

Answers—Unit A

Matching

1. c	**14.** d		
2. i	**15.** l		
3. o	**16.** g		
4. e	**17.** t		
5. v	**18.** x		
6. z	**19.** h		
7. a	**20.** y		
8. u	**21.** p		
9. q	**22.** w		
10. r	**23.** s		
11. b	**24.** k		
12. n	**25.** m		
13. j	**26.** f		

Outline

1. C	**15.** E
2. D	**16.** K
3. G	**17.** T
4. H	**18.** X
5. I	**19.** AC
6. N	**20.** B
7. S	**21.** F
8. U	**22.** L
9. V	**23.** M
10. W	**24.** O
11. Z	**25.** P
12. AA	**26.** Q
13. AB	**27.** R
14. A	**28.** Y

Multiple Choice

1. a	**18.** c
2. b	**19.** d
3. c	**20.** b
4. d	**21.** d
5. c	**22.** d
6. b	**23.** b
7. c	**24.** a
8. b	**25.** a
9. b	**26.** d
10. a	**27.** b
11. c	**28.** c
12. a	**29.** d
13. a	**30.** a
14. c	**31.** d
15. d	**32.** a
16. d	**33.** c
17. b	**34.** d

Activities

Labyrinth

1. G
2. A
3. B
4. F
5. E
6. C
7. D

Cross Section of Cochlea

1. G
2. H
3. N
4. M
5. D
6. A
7. L
8. I
9. K
10. J
11. E
12. F
13. P
14. C
15. B
16. O

UNIT B: NOISE

Background

Some estimates show that for several years the level of noise in the environment increased by as much as a decibel a year. Since no noise in nature can threaten human hearing without being infinitely more dangerous to physical safety, it is humankind that has visited this modern epidemic upon itself. In addition to interfering with communication, causing or increasing hearing loss, and causing nervous disorders, excessive noise has been linked to a number of physical and psychological diseases and decreased life expectancy. Noise-induced hearing losses may be of gradual or sudden onset, the latter sometimes referred to as acoustic trauma. The audiogram typical of a noise-induced hearing loss shows the greatest deficit in the 3000 to 6000 Hz range, often showing recovery of hearing in the higher frequencies; hence, the term *acoustic trauma notch*. Those hearing losses that improve over time have been called temporary threshold shifts (TTSs), and those that do not improve have been called permanent threshold shifts (PTSs). The audiologist must try to discover if noise is a factor in a patient's hearing loss and then help, by counseling, to find ways of preventing progression of the loss. Many audiologists are active in the industrial, military, legal, and political arenas, where debates about noise continue to be waged.

Objectives

1. You should know and understand the terms in the matching exercise.
2. You should be able to fill in the outline, selecting items from the list provided.
3. You should know the factors in the environment that produce dangerous noise levels.
4. You should know some strategies for dealing with patients who are exposed to high noise levels, including counseling techniques and the fitting of hearing protectors.
5. You should be able to answer the multiple-choice questions on the subject of noise.

Matching

Match the term from the box on the right with its definition

Definition

1. _____ Noise-induced hearing loss associated with sudden onset of intense noise

2. _____ A device that measures the intensity of noise over a period of time

3. _____ A federal agency designed to oversee the preservation of health and safety in the workplace

4. _____ Noise analysis with a sound-level meter that filters the sounds into narrow bands of 1 octave

5. _____ A reversible loss of hearing caused by intense noise

6. _____ Guidelines for avoiding noise-induced hearing loss that include noise intensity and time of exposure

7. _____ An irreversible loss of hearing caused by intense noise

8. _____ Any unwanted signal

Term

a. Acoustic trauma
b. Damage-risk criteria
c. Noise
d. Noise dosimeter
e. Octave-band analysis
f. OSHA
g. Permanent threshold shift
h. Temporary threshold shift

Outline

Noise

Auditory Effects

1. ____
2. ____
3. ____
4. ____
5. ____

Nonauditory Effects

6. ____
7. ____
8. ____
9. ____

Causes

10. ____
11. ____
12. ____

Measurement

13. ____
14. ____
15. ____

Damage-Risk Criteria

16. ____
17. ____

Agencies and Laws

18. ____
19. ____
20. ____
21. ____

Protection

22. ____
23. ____

Hearing Conservation

24. ____
25. ____

Select From

A. Acoustic trauma notch
B. Audiometric monitoring
C. EPA
D. Gunfire
E. Illness
F. Industry
G. Machinery
H. Muffs
I. Nervous disorders
J. NIOSH
K. Noise abatement
L. Noise dosimeter
M. Noise exposure time
N. Noise intensity
O. Noise survey
P. OSHA
Q. PTS
R. Plugs
S. Property damage
T. Psychological disorders
U. Sensorineural hearing loss
V. Speech interference
W. Sound-level meter
X. TTS
Y. Walsh-Healey Act

Multiple Choice

1. The drop in high-frequency hearing sensitivity secondary to sudden noise exposure is often called
   a. anacusis
   b. Carhart notch
   c. otosclerosis
   d. acoustic trauma notch
2. An irreversible impairment of hearing secondary to intense noise exposure is called
   a. permanent threshold shift
   b. conductive hypacusis
   c. temporary threshold shift
   d. anacusis
3. Many patients with noise-induced hearing loss report tinnitus in the frequency area of
   a. 250 Hz
   b. 500 Hz
   c. 4000 Hz
   d. 10,000 Hz
4. Sounds that produce a noise-induced hearing loss may be
   a. uncomfortably loud
   b. painful
   c. not uncomfortably loud
   d. all of the above
5. When the A scale of a sound-level meter is used, there is
   a. maximum deemphasis of the low frequencies
   b. moderate deemphasis of the high frequencies
   c. slight deemphasis of the high frequencies
   d. equal emphasis on all frequencies
6. Damage-risk criteria include the
   a. spectrum of the noise
   b. intensity of the noise
   c. duration of exposure
   d. all of the above
7. Maximum attenuation of noise is accomplished with
   a. acoustic earplugs in the ears
   b. fingers in the ears
   c. tragus pushed into the ear canal
   d. hands placed over the ears
8. Cases in which hearing thresholds improve after an initial impairment from excessive noise are called
   a. temporary threshold shift
   b. permanent threshold shift
   c. conductive hypacusis
   d. anacusis

9. The first federal act placing limits on noise levels allowable in workplaces doing government contract work was called
   a. ANSI
   b. ASA Act
   c. Walsh-Healey Act
   d. EPA Act

10. The filter setting used for most noise measurements on sound-level meters is the
   a. A scale
   b. B scale
   c. C scale
   d. D scale

11. Nonauditory effects of noise include
   a. property damage
   b. disease
   c. nervous conditions
   d. all of the above

12. A hunter who consistently fires a rifle from the right shoulder would be expected to have
   a. a greater loss in the right ear
   b. a greater loss in the left ear
   c. equal loss in both ears
   d. none of the above

Answers—Unit B

Matching	*Outline*	*Multiple Choice*
1. a	**1.** A	**1.** d
2. d	**2.** Q	**2.** a
3. f	**3.** U	**3.** c
4. e	**4.** V	**4.** d
5. h	**5.** X	**5.** a
6. b	**6.** E	**6.** d
7. g	**7.** I	**7.** c
8. c	**8.** S	**8.** a
	9. T	**9.** c
	10. D	**10.** a
	11. F	**11.** d
	12. G	**12.** b
	13. L	
	14. O	
	15. W	
	16. M	
	17. N	
	18. C	
	19. J	
	20. P	
	21. Y	
	22. H	
	23. R	
	24. B	
	25. K	

12 The Auditory Nerve and Central Auditory Pathways

Background

The nerve fibers arising from the cristae of the semicircular canals and the maculae of the utricle and saccule form the vestibular branch of the auditory (VIIIth cranial) nerve. The nerve fibers from the cochlea emerge from the modiolus to form the cochlear branch of the VIIIth nerve, which is primarily afferent (sensory) in that it carries impulses from the cochlea to the brain. It is also efferent (inhibitory), carrying impulses back to the inner ear by way of the olivocochlear bundle. The VIIIth nerve ascends to the brainstem through the internal auditory canal, from which the cochlear branch goes to a series of ipsilateral (same side of the brain) and contralateral (opposite side of the brain) waystations on its way to Heschl's gyrus in the temporal lobe. There is tonotopicity in many of these waystations.

A variety of pathologies can interfere with the neural transmission of sound and an individual's ability to process speech. Lesions within the higher auditory pathways can produce subtle symptoms that may prove insensitive to routine audiological studies. Special procedures have been devised to evaluate central auditory disorders, but none has proven infallible, underlining the importance of a complete test battery approach to the evaluation of disorders beyond the cochlea.

Objectives

1. You should know and understand the terms in the matching exercise.
2. You should be able to fill in the outline, selecting items from the list provided.
3. You should be able to label the different parts of the auditory pathways in Figure 12.1.
4. You should be able to do the matching exercise.
5. You should be able to answer the multiple-choice questions and understand the anatomy of the central auditory system as well as causes of disorders that produce sensorineural hearing loss or auditory processing difficulties.

Matching

Match the term from the box on the right with its definition.

Definition

1. ____ The base of the brain where it connects to the spinal cord

2. ____ The gray matter on the surface of the brain

3. ____ That part of the central auditory pathway found in the midbrain

4. ____ The area of the brainstem that provides facilitation and inhibition of afferent stimuli

5. ____ The VIIIth cranial nerve

6. ____ The area of the pons that connects the ventral cochlear nucleus with the lateral lemniscus on the other side of the brain

7. ____ The bridge connecting the two hemispheres of the brain at its base

8. ____ Anatomical arrangement according to the best frequency of stimulation

9. ____ The area of the brain receiving fibers from the ipsilateral cochlea by way of the VIIIth cranial nerve

10. ____ Part of the auditory pathway receiving fibers from the cochlear nucleus

11. ____ The theory that nerve units fire their entire electrical charge when their threshold of stimulation is reached

12. ____ The superior temporal gyrus of the brain

13. ____ Fibers in the temporal cortex received from the medial geniculate body

14. ____ The addition of energy to stimulate a nerve unit

15. ____ The part of the brain above the pons and medulla that is responsible for equilibrium

Terms

a. All-or-none
b. Auditory nerve
c. Auditory radiations
d. Brainstem
e. Central nervous system
f. Cerebellopontine angle
g. Cerebellum
h. Cerebral cortex
i. Cochlear nucleus
j. Commissure
k. Decussation
l. Excitation
m. Extra-axial
n. Glia
o. Heschl's gyrus
p. Inferior colliculus
q. Inhibition
r. Integration
s. Internal auditory canal
t. Intra-axial
u. Lateral lemniscus
v. Medial geniculate body
w. Obscure auditory dysfunction
x. Olivocochlear bundle
y. Pons
z. Reticular formation
aa. Superior olivary complex
ab. Thalamus
ac. Tonotopicity
ad. Trapezoid body

Definition

16. _____ The crossing over of nerve fibers from one side of the brain to the other

17. _____ The passage from the inner ear to the brainstem containing the two branches of the VIIIth nerve, facial nerve, and internal auditory artery

18. _____ Arresting or restraining a neural impulse

19. _____ The portion of the auditory pathway running from the cochlear nucleus to the inferior colliculus and medial geniculate body

20. _____ A group of fibers in the brainstem that provides inhibition to the cochlear nucleus and cochlea

21. _____ The brain and spinal cord

22. _____ Connective tissue in the brain

23. _____ Within the brainstem

24. _____ The combining of different neural functions to facilitate a process

25. _____ The area in the brain base that communicates with the cortex

26. _____ The last subcortical relay station, found in the thalamus

27. _____ The junction at the base of the brain where the cerebellum, medulla, and pons communicate

28. _____ Outside of the brainstem

29. _____ Specialized nerve fibers that connect the hemispheres of the brain

30. _____ Decreased hearing abilities, primarily in adverse listening conditions, in the absence of identifiable peripheral pathology

Terms

a. All-or-none
b. Auditory nerve
c. Auditory radiations
d. Brainstem
e. Central nervous system
f. Cerebellopontine angle
g. Cerebellum
h. Cerebral cortex
i. Cochlear nucleus
j. Commissure
k. Decussation
l. Excitation
m. Extra-axial
n. Glia
o. Heschl's gyrus
p. Inferior colliculus
q. Inhibition
r. Integration
s. Internal auditory canal
t. Intra-axial
u. Lateral lemniscus
v. Medial geniculate body
w. Obscure auditory dysfunction
x. Olivocochlear bundle
y. Pons
z. Reticular formation
aa. Superior olivary complex
ab. Thalamus
ac. Tonotopicity
ad. Trapezoid body

Outline

The Auditory Nerve and Central Pathways
Anatomy of the VIIIth Nerve

1. ____
2. ____
3. ____
4. ____

Waystations in the Brainstem

5. ____
6. ____
7. ____
8. ____
9. ____

First-Order Neurons

10. ____

Second-Order Neurons

11. ____

Waystations in the Midbrain

12. ____
13. ____

Fibers in the Cortex

14. ____
15. ____

Disorders

16. ____
17. ____
18. ____
19. ____
20. ____
21. ____

Evaluative Measures

22. ____
23. ____
24. ____
25. ____

Select From

A. Aging
B. Auditory radiations
C. Cochlea to cochlear nucleus
D. Cochlear branch
E. Course from the cochlear nucleus
F. Dichotic digits test
G. Dorsal cochlear nucleus
H. Heschl's gyrus
I. Inferior colliculus
J. Internal auditory canal
K. Lateral lemniscus
L. Medial geniculate body
M. Multiple sclerosis
N. Myelin sheath
O. Neuritis
P. Screening test for auditory processing disorders (SCAN)
Q. Staggered spondaic word (SSW) test
R. Superior olivary complex
S. Time compressed speech
T. Trapezoid body
U. Trauma
V. Tumors
W. Ventral cochlear nucleus
X. Vestibular branch
Y. Viral infections

Activity

Label the parts of the ascending auditory pathways in Figure 12.1, selecting the terms from the list provided. Compare your labels with those at the end of this unit.

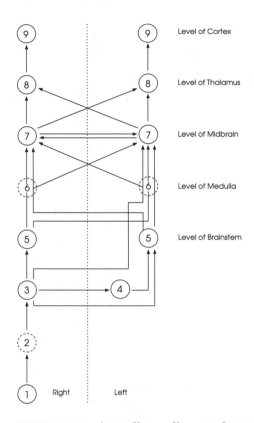

FIGURE 12.1.   Ascending auditory pathways.

Label		*Term*
1. _____		**A.** Auditory cortex
2. _____		**B.** Auditory nerve (cochlear branch)
3. _____		**C.** Cochlea
4. _____		**D.** Cochlear nucleus (dorsal and ventral)
5. _____		**E.** Inferior colliculus
6. _____		**F.** Lateral lemniscus
7. _____		**G.** Medial geniculate body
8. _____		**H.** Superior olivary complex
9. _____		**I.** Trapezoid body

Multiple Choice

1. To test for central auditory disorders in a patient with normal hearing sensitivity, the audiologist will
   a. increase the extrinsic redundancy
   b. decrease the extrinsic redundancy
   c. increase the intrinsic redundancy
   d. decrease the intrinsic redundancy
2. The last subcortical relay station for auditory impulses is the
   a. inferior colliculus
   b. lateral lemniscus
   c. cochlear nucleus
   d. medial geniculate body
3. The auditory nerve is number
   a. V
   b. VI
   c. VII
   d. VIII
4. The efferent auditory system is designed for
   a. control of muscular activity
   b. feedback to lower auditory centers
   c. feed through to higher auditory centers
   d. work only at high intensities
5. The reticular formation is thought to aid in
   a. facilitation
   b. inhibition
   c. both of the above
   d. neither a nor b
6. The eyeblink is mediated through
   a. superior olivary complex
   b. inferior colliculus
   c. lateral lemniscus
   d. cochlear nucleus
7. Lesions of the central auditory nervous system include
   a. tumors
   b. degenerative diseases
   c. trauma
   d. all of the above
8. Acoustic neuromas usually form
   a. on the facial nerve
   b. on the cochlear branch of the auditory nerve
   c. on the vestibular branch of the auditory nerve
   d. in the superior olivary complex

9. Crossover points uniting symmetrical portions of the two halves of the brain are called
   a. tonotopic
   b. decussations
   c. neurons
   d. none of the above

10. Fibers cross from the left cochlear nucleus to the right cochlear nucleus via the
    a. trapezoid body
    b. superior olivary complex
    c. lateral lemniscus
    d. inferior colliculus

11. The cochlear nucleus is divided into
    a. superior and inferior portions
    b. left and right portions
    c. dorsal and ventral portions
    d. none of the above

12. Impulses are transmitted from the lower brainstem to the inferior colliculus by way of the
    a. lateral lemniscus
    b. medial geniculate body
    c. thalamus
    d. auditory radiations

13. Heschl's gyrus is located in the
    a. brainstem
    b. midbrain
    c. thalamus
    d. cortex

14. Given a patient with a lesion of the left auditory nerve, a rollover on a PI/PB function would be expected in
    a. the right ear
    b. the left ear
    c. both ears
    d. neither ear

15. Given a patient with a lesion of the left temporal lobe, a rollover on a PI/PB function would be expected in
    a. the right ear
    b. the left ear
    c. both ears
    d. neither ear

16. On auditory brainstem response (ABR) testing a patient with a tumor of the left auditory nerve would be expected to show
    a. longer latency to wave V in the right ear than in the left ear
    b. longer latency to wave V in the left ear than in the right ear
    c. the same latency for both ears
    d. none of the above

17. Otoacoustic emissions in cases of acoustic neuroma are expected to be
    a. absent in the impaired ear, present in the normal ear
    b. present in the impaired ear, absent in the normal ear
    c. absent in the impaired ear, absent in the normal ear
    d. present in the impaired ear, present in the normal ear
18. A screening measure for retrocochlear lesion utilizing speech recognition measures repeated at a variety of sensation levels is
    a. masking-level difference
    b. Heschl's speech score
    c. performance-intensity function
    d. staggered spondaic word test
19. A disorder that creates decreased hearing abilities in noise in the absence of identifiable peripheral pathology is called
    a. auditory neuropathy
    b. obscure auditory dysfunction
    c. reticular nucleitis
    d. acoustic neuritis
20. Difficulty in language learning arising from a decrease in the size of neurons in the central auditory nervous system may be the result of
    a. masking-level differences
    b. multiple sclerosis
    c. neurofibromatosis
    d. minimal auditory deficiency syndrome

Answers

Matching	*Outline*	*Activity*	*Multiple Choice*
1. d	**1.** D	**1.** C	**1.** b
2. h	**2.** I	**2.** B	**2.** d
3. p	**3.** M	**3.** D	**3.** d
4. z	**4.** T	**4.** I	**4.** b
5. b	**5.** F	**5.** H	**5.** c
6. ad	**6.** J	**6.** F	**6.** a
7. y	**7.** O	**7.** E	**7.** d
8. ac	**8.** P	**8.** G	**8.** c
9. i	**9.** S	**9.** A	**9.** b
10. c	**10.** C		**10.** a
11. a	**11.** E		**11.** c
12. o	**12.** H		**12.** a
13. c	**13.** K		**13.** d
14. l	**14.** B		**14.** b
15. g	**15.** G		**15.** a
16. k	**16.** A		**16.** b
17. s	**17.** L		**17.** a
18. q	**18.** M		**18.** c
19. u	**19.** Q		**19.** b
20. m	**20.** R		**20.** d
21. e	**21.** U		
22. n	**22.** F		
23. t	**23.** P		
24. r	**24.** Q		
25. ab	**25.** S		
26. v			
27. f			
28. m			
29. j			
30. ae			

CHAPTER

13 Nonorganic Hearing Loss

Background

Some patients seen for hearing evaluations may feign or exaggerate a hearing loss. Terms that describe this behavior, which may be on a conscious or unconscious level, include nonorganic hearing loss, pseudohypacusis, malingering, psychogenic hearing loss, functional hearing loss, conversion deafness, and a host of others. It is the responsibility of the audiologist to recognize nonorganic hearing loss and to determine the patient's true hearing status, albeit without the patient's cooperation. Some tests are quantitative; that is, they provide fairly precise information about a patient's true organic thresholds; other tests are merely qualitative and provide evidence of nonorganic hearing loss. After diagnosis comes the sometimes more formidable task of patient management and, when indicated, appropriate referral.

Objectives

1. You should know and understand the terms in the matching exercise.
2. You should be able to fill in the outline, selecting items from the list provided.
3. You should know which tests are appropriate for different kinds and degrees of nonorganic hearing loss.
4. You should know the equipment that is required for different tests for nonorganic hearing loss.
5. You should be able to answer the multiple-choice questions on nonorganic hearing loss.

Matching

Match the term from the box on the right with its definition.

Definition

1. _____ A test for nonorganic hearing loss utilizing spondees and broadband noise

2. _____ The willful act of feigning a hearing loss or other disorder

3. _____ Early auditory evoked potentials

4. _____ Nonorganic hearing loss presumably at the unconscious level

5. _____ A test based on the fact that people speak more loudly when they hear a loud noise

6. _____ A term for claimed hearing loss that is not explainable in terms of organic pathology

7. _____ A synonym for nonorganic hearing loss

8. _____ A test for nonorganic hearing loss involving a delay between the time a patient taps a finger or utters a word and the time the sound is heard

Term

a. Auditory brainstem response
b. Delayed auditory feedback
c. Doerfler-Stewart test
d. Lombard test
e. Malingering
f. Nonorganic hearing loss
g. Pseudohypacusis
h. Psychogenic hearing loss

Outline

Nonorganic Hearing Loss
Terminology

1. ____
2. ____
3. ____
4. ____
5. ____
6. ____

Test for Unilateral Nonorganic Hearing Loss

7. ____

General Tests for Nonorganic Hearing Loss

8. ____
9. ____
10. ____
11. ____
12. ____

Select From

A. Auditory brainstem response
B. Conversion deafness
C. Delayed auditory feedback
D. Doerfler-Stewart test
E. Functional hearing loss
F. Lombard test
G. Malingering
H. Nonorganic hearing loss
I. Pseudohypacusis
J. Psychogenic hearing loss
K. Stenger test
L. VIST

Multiple Choice

1. When a nonorganic hearing loss is suspected, the audiologist may best increase cooperation by
   a. confronting the patient
   b. counseling the patient about his or her ethical responsibilities
   c. shifting the blame to the examiner
   d. insisting on greater attention to the tests
2. A nonorganic hearing loss of an unconscious nature is called
   a. sinistrosis
   b. psychogenic hearing loss
   c. nonorganic hearing loss
   d. malingering
3. The following is *not* an alerting sign for nonorganic hearing loss
   a. source of referral
   b. behavior during the interview/case history
   c. elevated acoustic reflexes
   d. performance on routine tests
4. The problem with most tests for nonorganic hearing loss is that they are
   a. nonqualitative
   b. nonquantitative
   c. too qualitative
   d. easy to beat
5. The following test for nonorganic hearing loss is limited to unilateral losses
   a. pure-tone delayed auditory feedback
   b. Stenger test
   c. Doerfler-Stewart test
   d. Lombard test
6. The following is a typical finding with nonorganic hearing loss
   a. SRT worse than PTA
   b. sensorineural loss with absent acoustic reflexes
   c. conductive loss with absent acoustic reflexes
   d. lack of cross-hearing in unilateral loss
7. The Lombard test can be done as part of
   a. delayed-speech feedback
   b. Doerfler-Stewart test
   c. VIST
   d. Stenger test
8. In nonorganic hearing loss the general finding is
   a. SRT = PTA
   b. SRT lower (better) than PTA
   c. SRT higher (poorer) than PTA
   d. SRT = SDT

9. The following test gives the best estimate of threshold
   a. pure-tone DAF
   b. Stenger test
   c. Doerfler-Stewart test
   d. Lombard test
10. Elevation of vocal output in the presence of noise is called the
    a. Lombard voice reflex
    b. paracusis willisi
    c. Doerfler-Stewart effect
    d. Stenger effect
11. Malingering can be proven only if
    a. the patient admits it
    b. ABR reveals normal hearing
    c. the Stenger is positive
    d. otoacoustic emissions are present
12. Nonorganic hearing loss involving a deliberate act is called
    a. hysterical deafness
    b. psychogenic hearing loss
    c. nonorganic hearing loss
    d. malingering
13. Threshold can probably best be determined on a nonorganic hearing loss patient showing bilateral hearing loss with the
    a. VIST
    b. ABR
    c. Doerfler-Stewart test
    d. Stenger test
14. The minimum contralateral interference level is designed to
    a. screen for nonorganicity on the Stenger
    b. indicate precise threshold on the Stenger
    c. modify the Stenger
    d. approximate threshold on the Stenger
15. Key tapping is used with
    a. pure-tone DAF
    b. speech DAF
    c. LOCK test
    d. Békésy audiometry
16. The latest addition to the battery of tests for nonorganic hearing loss is
    a. otoacoustic emissions
    b. ABR
    c. Stenger test
    d. Lombard test

Answers

Matching	*Outline*	*Multiple Choice*
1. d	**1.** C	**1.** c
2. g	**2.** E	**2.** b
3. a	**3.** A	**3.** c
4. e	**4.** H	**4.** b
5. j	**5.** D	**5.** b
6. f	**6.** F	**6.** d
7. i	**7.** G	**7.** a
8. b	**8.** B	**8.** b
9. h	**9.** C	**9.** a
10. c	**10.** D	**10.** a
	11. F	**11.** a
	12. L	**12.** d
		13. b
		14. d
		15. a
		16. a

14 Amplification/Sensory Systems

Background

As the hearing aid evolved from acoustic amplifiers such as ear trumpets into the electronic era, research has focused on miniaturization and improved sound quality. The current infusion of microprocessing techniques into the design characteristics and the selection and verification procedures for hearing aids is bringing about a new revolution in this most important aspect of audiological rehabilitation. The hearing aid is essentially a one-way transmission system containing a microphone as an input transducer, a miniature loudspeaker as an output transducer, and stages of amplification with volume control and signal shaping and processing between these two. The system is powered by a small battery. Although there is some limited need today for bone-conduction receivers, most instruments generate air-conduction signals. Acoustic characteristics of hearing aids are usually described in terms of their saturation sound-pressure level (SSPL, the maximum power output that can be delivered regardless of the strength of the input signal), acoustic gain (the difference in decibels between the input and output sound-pressure levels), and the frequency response (range and output of frequencies amplified). No modern audiology clinic should be without a hearing-aid testing system that can measure the characteristics of hearing aids, including their distortion products. Although no single procedure for evaluating and selecting the "best" hearing aids to suit an individual patient is agreed upon, the present trend is toward dispensing the selected instruments directly to the patient rather than writing a prescription for a particular make, model, and set of internal and external settings, as was popular only a short time ago. It is hoped that the days of selecting hearing aids from mail-order catalogues or drug or department stores are nearly over and that hearing aids can be offered to patients as part of a larger package of auditory (re)training, speech reading, hearing-aid orientation, and counseling.

The use of hearing aids alone may not always provide the full benefit a patient's hearing deficit may require. To augment the benefit derived from hearing aids, a variety of hearing assistance technologies has been developed. For some patients, cochlear reserve is so low that auditory amplification provides no measurable improvement. These patients may be assisted through instruments that provide tactile stimulation on the skin's surface in response to acoustic stimuli, or instrumentation to provide direct electrical stimulation to the auditory nerve through cochlear implants.

Objectives

1. You should know and understand the terms in the matching exercise.
2. You should be able to fill in the outline, selecting items from the list provided.
3. You should know and be able to identify the components of a hearing aid.
4. You should understand the implications of assistive listening devices.
5. You should be able to answer the multiple-choice questions about hearing instruments.

Matching

Match the term from the box on the right with its definition.

Definition

1. _____ A device surgically placed in the inner ear for persons with profound hearing loss

2. _____ The squeal that occurs when sound that is amplified and fed through the speaker of a hearing aid is picked up again by the microphone and reamplified

3. _____ An amplification system that stores and processes the input signal as sets of binary digits that represent frequency, intensity, and temporal patterns of the signal

4. _____ A device that amplifies sound and delivers it to the surface of the skin so that the different patterns of vibration can be felt

5. _____ Measurements made of sound-pressure level in the ear canal that show the performance characteristics of a hearing aid

6. _____ Signaling or alerting devices, in addition to hearing aids, that assist individuals with a hearing loss

7. _____ An electromagnetic device in a hearing aid that allows the user to bypass the microphone when talking on the telephone

8. _____ Hearing aids worn in both ears

9. _____ The highest sound pressure that can emit from a hearing aid regardless of the input intensity

10. _____ The custom-made device, usually made of plastic, that couples a hearing aid to the ear

11. _____ A system for limiting the sound intensity emitted by a hearing aid by using electronic feedback circuits

Term

a. Acoustic feedback
b. Acoustic gain
c. Automatic gain control
d. Binaural hearing aids
e. Cochlear implants
f. Compression amplification
g. Digital hearing aid
h. Earmold
i. Frequency response
j. Harmonic distortion
k. Hearing assistance technologies / Assistive listening devices
l. Real ear insertion gain (REIR)
m. Probe tube
n. Real-ear measurements
o. Reference test gain
p. Saturation sound-pressure level
q. Telecoil
r. Vibrotactile hearing aid

Definition

12. _____ Connection to the space between the medial end of an ear mold or hearing aid casing and the tympanic membrane so that a sound in that space can be measured

13. _____ The range from the lowest to the highest frequency amplified by a hearing aid

14. _____ A specified average increase of the intensity of a sound produced by a hearing aid as measured in a hearing aid test box

15. _____ The difference, in decibels, between the input intensity and the output intensity of a hearing aid

16. _____ Distortion in a hearing aid produced by the generation of overtones

17. _____ Another term for automatic gain control

18. _____ Hearing aid gain obtained through probe-microphone measures

Term

a. Acoustic feedback
b. Acoustic gain
c. Automatic gain control
d. Binaural hearing aids
e. Cochlear implants
f. Compression amplification
g. Digital hearing aid
h. Earmold
i. Frequency response
j. Harmonic distortion
k. Hearing assistance technologies / Assistive listening devices
l. Real ear insertion gain (REIR)
m. Probe tube
n. Real-ear measurements
o. Reference test gain
p. Saturation sound-pressure level
q. Telecoil
r. Vibrotactile hearing aid

Outline

Hearing Aids
Types

1. ____
2. ____
3. ____
4. ____
5. ____
6. ____
7. ____
8. ____
9. ____

Characteristics

10. ____
11. ____
12. ____
13. ____
14. ____
15. ____

Components

16. ____
17. ____
18. ____
19. ____
20. ____
21. ____
22. ____
23. ____
24. ____

Select From

A. Air conduction
B. Amplifier
C. Battery
D. Behind-the-ear
E. Body-worn
F. Bone conduction
G. Completely in-the-canal
H. Cord
I. CROS
J. Digital processor
K. Earmold
L. Eyeglass
M. Frequency response
N. Gain
O. Harmonic distortion
P. Intermodulation distortion
Q. In-the-canal
R. In-the-ear
S. Microphone
T. Peak clipping
U. SSPL
V. Telephone pickup (telecoil)
W. Tone control
X. Volume control

Multiple Choice

1. The maximum sound-pressure level emitted from the receiver of a hearing aid, regardless of its input level is called
   a. acoustic gain
   b. SSPL
   c. frequency response
   d. distortion

2. The difference, in decibels, between the input and the output SPL of a hearing aid is its
   a. acoustic gain
   b. SSPL
   c. frequency response
   d. distortion

3. A sweep frequency audio oscillator is used to determine a hearing aid's
   a. acoustic output
   b. SSPL
   c. frequency response
   d. distortion

4. Lack of sound coming from a hearing aid may be caused by
   a. occluded earmold
   b. twisted tubing
   c. a broken receiver
   d. all of the above

5. Acoustic feedback will not be caused by
   a. a loosely fitting earmold
   b. a twisted cord
   c. a loose connection between earmold and receiver
   d. an improperly inserted earmold

6. Weak but audible sound coming from a hearing aid will not be caused by a
   a. partially obstructed earmold
   b. weak battery
   c. switch set to "telephone" setting
   d. partially obstructed tubing

7. The input transducer of a hearing aid is its
   a. battery
   b. microphone
   c. loudspeaker
   d. volume control

8. "Ceramic," "magnetic," "dynamic," and "electret" are different kinds of
   a. loudspeakers
   b. hearing aids
   c. microphones
   d. volume controls

9. Deemphasis of different portions of the frequency response of a hearing aid may be accomplished by
   a. earmold modification
   b. internal tone adjustments
   c. changing receivers
   d. all of the above
10. Bone-conduction hearing aids are usually reserved for patients who have
    a. sensorineural hearing loss
    b. conductive hearing losses caused by otosclerosis
    c. conductive hearing losses with chronic ear drainage
    d. mixed hearing losses without chronic ear drainage
11. Acoustic feedback problems with hearing aids will not be lessened by
    a. cupping a hand behind the aided ear
    b. increasing the distance from microphone to receiver
    c. fabricating a tighter earmold
    d. replacing a cracked or damaged earmold tubing
12. Binaural amplification will
    a. improve hearing in noise
    b. improve localization abilities
    c. decrease the effects of sensory deprivation
    d. all of the above
13. Persons with total unilateral hearing losses are sometimes helped by a hearing aid called
    a. CROS
    b. IROS
    c. NITTS
    d. ROSS
14. Cochlear implants are
    a. totally placed within the middle ear
    b. limited to use with children who have prelingistic hearing loss
    c. effective for some recipients for telephone conversations
    d. none of the above

Answers

Matching	*Outline*	*Multiple Choice*
1. e	**1.** A	**1.** b
2. a	**2.** D	**2.** a
3. g	**3.** E	**3.** c
4. r	**4.** F	**4.** d
5. n	**5.** G	**5.** b
6. k	**6.** I	**6.** c
7. q	**7.** L	**7.** b
8. d	**8.** Q	**8.** c
9. p	**9.** R	**9.** d
10. h	**10.** M	**10.** c
11. c	**11.** N	**11.** a
12. m	**12.** O	**12.** d
13. i	**13.** P	**13.** a
14. o	**14.** T	**14.** c
15. b	**15.** U	
16. j	**16.** B	
17. f	**17.** C	
18. l	**18.** H	
	19. J	
	20. S	
	21. R	
	22. V	
	23. W	
	24. X	

15 Audiological (Re)Habilitation

UNIT A: APPROACHES TO REHABILITATION

Background

All the diagnostic audiological information gathered on a patient is useless unless it translates into some form of constructive action that helps the patient to communicate. Medical or surgical reversal of hearing loss is preferable, but when this is impossible or when the treatment does not result in sufficient functional hearing, steps must be taken to improve the patient's communicative abilities by utilizing residual hearing. High on the list of measures to be considered is the selection and training in the use of proper hearing aids if this is feasible. Other measures include auditory (re)training; speechreading; and, foremost, education and counseling of patients and their families regarding the implications of hearing loss. Although drill work in speechreading or discrimination of sounds is still widely practiced, it is considered by many clinicians not to be the most effectual means of audiological rehabilitation for many persons. Many clinicians today construct their therapy around hearing-handicap scales, completed by the patient, to help to judge the kinds of communicative difficulties that are experienced. Proper audiological rehabilitation is the culmination of the efforts of the clinical audiologist.

Objectives

1. You should know and understand the terms in the matching exercise.
2. You should be able to fill in the outline, selecting items from the list provided.
3. You should try to understand some of the feelings of many patients with hearing disabilities so that these may be dealt with more efficiently.
4. You should understand the basic principles of speechreading training.
5. You should understand the basic principles of auditory training.
6. You should understand the basic principles of patient counseling.
7. You should be able to answer the multiple-choice questions.

Matching

Match the term from the box on the right with its definition.

Definition

1. _____ A class of closely related speech sounds

2. _____ The production of speech as it appears on the lips

3. _____ The reeducation of individuals who have lost their hearing in listening for specific auditory cues

4. _____ The use of facial cues to determine the words of a speaker

5. _____ The recording of all background information related to a hearing loss

6. _____ A ringing or other sound heard in the ears or the head

7. _____ Any part of a word that conveys meaning

8. _____ Group instruction to help surmount variables within the environment, or poor speaker or listener habits, that impede successful communication

9. _____ Therapy to maintain clear articulation when auditory feedback of speech production has been decreased by postlinguistic hearing loss

Term

a. Auditory retraining
b. Hearing therapy
c. History taking
d. Morpheme
e. Phoneme
f. Speech conservation
g. Speechreading
h. Visime
i. Tinnitus

Outline

Audiological Rehabilitation
Speechreading
1. _____
2. _____
3. _____
4. _____

Auditory Training
5. _____
6. _____
7. _____
8. _____

Counseling
9. _____
10. _____
11. _____
12. _____
13. _____
14. _____
15. _____

Select From
A. Adjustment to hearing aids
B. Analytical methods
C. Combined with residual hearing
D. Communication guidelines
E. Coping strategies
F. Group counseling
G. Individual counseling
H. Hearing aid orientation
I. Social strategies
J. Word recognition in noise
K. Word recognition in quiet
L. Synthetic methods
M. Support groups
N. Tolerance for loud sounds
O. Visible phonemes

Multiple Choice

1. Important to a course in auditory training is the teaching of
   a. discrimination among speech sounds
   b. discrimination of speech sounds from nonspeech sounds
   c. discrimination of sound from silence
   d. all of the above
2. Speech detection implies
   a. sensing whether a sound is present
   b. the nature of a particular sound
   c. discrimination among speech sounds
   d. all of the above
3. Identification of speech sounds by a patient may be indicated by
   a. repeating the sound
   b. pointing to a picture or item
   c. writing down what was heard
   d. all of the above
4. Auditory retraining is a term used to denote that
   a. the hearing loss was adventitious
   b. the hearing loss was congenital
   c. the hearing loss was inherited
   d. all of the above
5. Audiological rehabilitation is usually most difficult for a patient with a moderate hearing loss that is
   a. conductive
   b. mixed
   c. sensorineural
   d. unilateral
6. The term *habilitation* is usually used when describing work with
   a. very young children
   b. teenagers
   c. adults
   d. the elderly
7. Aural rehabilitation often involves teaching adults to
   a. utilize contextual cues in speech
   b. make reasonable guesses
   c. predict language patterns
   d. all of the above
8. The least difficult listening situation for the new hearing-aid wearer is
   a. understanding in quiet places
   b. understanding in noisy places
   c. understanding rapid speakers
   d. understanding unusual vocabulary

9. Patients wearing hearing aids can learn to improve the signal-to-noise ratio when listening in a noisy place by
   a. raising the volume of the hearing aids
   b. moving closer to the speaker
   c. asking the speaker to talk louder
   d. b and c

10. A basic assumption that may be made when hearing aids are provided to a small child is that
    a. speech will be clearer
    b. speech will be louder
    c. speech will be louder and clearer
    d. visual cues are unnecessary

11. A first step in an audiological habilitation program with a small child is sound
    a. repetition
    b. awareness
    c. discrimination
    d. production

12. Although there is some disagreement, most clinicians believe that audiological habilitation should include
    a. visual cues alone
    b. auditory cues alone
    c. visual and auditory cues combined
    d. none of the above

13. Of the more than 40 phonemes used in English discourse, approximately _____ are clearly visible
    a. 90 percent
    b. 20 percent
    c. 33 percent
    d. 5 percent

14. Most difficult to speechread are
    a. vowels
    b. consonants
    c. words in context
    d. sentences

15. Many audiologists believe that speechreading ability
    a. can be taught equally to all patients
    b. is a talent possessed more by some people than by others
    c. is unimportant if properly fitted hearing aids are used
    d. is easily learned

16. The ability to speechread is affected by
    a. the available light
    b. distance from the speaker
    c. rate of the speech
    d. all of the above

17. It is important to teach visual memory when teaching speechreading because
    a. speech is usually not repeated
    b. speech is rapid
    c. speech sounds, once seen, cannot be reviewed
    d. all of the above
18. SHHH is an acronym for
    a. Silence Here for Hard of Hearing
    b. Still Have Hearing Handicap
    c. Self Help for Hard of Hearing People
    d. Should Holler for Hard of Hearing

Answers—Unit A

Matching	*Outline*	*Multiple Choice*
1. e	**1.** B	**1.** d
2. h	**2.** C	**2.** a
3. a	**3.** L	**3.** d
4. g	**4.** O	**4.** a
5. c	**5.** A	**5.** c
6. i	**6.** J	**6.** a
7. d	**7.** K	**7.** d
8. b	**8.** N	**8.** a
9. f	**9.** D	**9.** d
	10. E	**10.** b
	11. F	**11.** b
	12. G	**12.** c
	13. H	**13.** c
	14. I	**14.** a
	15. M	**15.** b
		16. d
		17. d
		18. c

UNIT B: EDUCATION OF CHILDREN WITH HEARING IMPAIRMENTS

Background

Children who are born with or acquire a hearing loss before they develop speech and language are said to be prelinguistically hearing impaired. If their hearing loss exceeds 70 dB HL, they cannot be expected to hear more than the loudest environmental sounds and will not develop spoken language or achieve a suitable education without special training and the use of amplification. If the loss exceeds 90 dB HL, even with amplification, the auditory channel alone will not suffice for their learning. The proper methods of educating children with a severe hearing handicap are not agreed upon, even among the most well-meaning experts. One group believes that the "deaf" should be considered as a group unto themselves with no attempt made to integrate them educationally into a hearing environment. These people are often committed to one of several forms of manual communication. The so-called "oralists" believe that children should be taught speech at all costs, taking maximum advantage of residual hearing through amplification, and should use no signs whatever. Still others believe in a combined approach of simultaneously speaking and signing. Regardless of the preferred method, there is universal agreement that the earlier the hearing loss is detected and steps taken toward educating the child, the better the prognosis for the development of language at an early age and the achievement of the highest possible educational attainment.

Objectives

1. You should know and understand the terms in the matching exercise.
2. You should be able to fill in the outline, selecting items from the list provided.
3. You should understand the methods, advantages, and disadvantages of the manual approaches to educating children with hearing impairments.
4. You should understand the methods, advantages, and disadvantages of the oral approaches to educating children with hearing impairments.
5. You should understand the methods, advantages, and disadvantages of the combined approaches to educating children with hearing impairments.
6. You should be able to answer the multiple-choice questions on pediatric management.

Matching

Match the term from the box on the right with its definition.

Definition

1. _____ The use of hand signs and facial and body movements in communicating with persons with a hearing impairment

2. _____ A method of manual communication that follows English word order but is relatively uncommon

3. _____ Writing in the air with the fingers to spell out words

4. _____ Using hand signs with specific signs for articles and verbs

5. _____ A unisensory approach to teaching children with severe hearing loss that relies solely on hearing

6. _____ A less than normally rigid system of signs

7. _____ Educating individuals with hearing impairment to maximize auditory cues, often utilizing drilling exercises

8. _____ Educating children in the least restrictive environment

9. _____ A multisensory approach to teaching speech

Term

a. American Sign Language
b. Auditory training
c. Auditory-verbal training
d. Aural/oral
e. Finger spelling
f. Linguistics of Visual English
g. Mainstreaming
h. Signing Essential English
i. Signing Exact English

Outline

Education of Children Who Are Hearing Impaired

Goals

1. ____
2. ____
3. ____
4. ____
5. ____

Assessment

6. ____
7. ____
8. ____
9. ____

Communication Skills

10. ____
11. ____
12. ____
13. ____

Communication Systems

14. ____
15. ____
16. ____
17. ____
18. ____
19. ____
20. ____
21. ____
22. ____

Select From

A. American Sign Language
B. Auditory global method
C. Auditory training
D. Educational achievement
E. Educational potential
F. Finger spelling
G. Integration into Deaf society
H. Integration into hearing society
I. Intelligence
J. Language
K. Language concepts
L. Linguistics of Visual English
M. Multisensory stimulation
N. Personality
O. Psychological potential
P. Seeing Essential English
Q. Signing Exact English
R. Social potential
S. Speech
T. Speechreading
U. Systematic sign language
V. Total communication

Multiple Choice

1. The sign system about which most information is known is
   a. ASL
   b. LOVE
   c. SEE1
   d. AMESLISH
2. All elements of English grammar may be included in
   a. LOVE
   b. SEE1
   c. finger spelling
   d. ASL
3. The least extensive sign system in terms of vocabulary is
   a. ASL
   b. LOVE
   c. SEE1
   d. SEE2
4. Signing and speaking simultaneously is called
   a. ASL
   b. total communication
   c. visual communication
   d. SEE3
5. A generic term describing hearing disability regardless of degree is
   a. hearing impaired
   b. hard of hearing
   c. deaf
   d. deafened
6. Children with hearing losses in the 70 to 90 dB HL range, without amplification, may be expected to
   a. have difficulty mainly with faint speech
   b. understand conversation at distances less than 5 feet
   c. understand speech only if speakers raise their voices
   d. identify loud sounds near the ear and perhaps a few vowel sounds
7. Given appropriate training and amplification, success may usually be achieved in regular schools by children with hearing losses up to
   a. 30 dB HL
   b. 50 dB HL
   c. 70 dB HL
   d. 90 dB HL
8. Early identification is most likely for a child with a hearing loss of
   a. 20 dB HL
   b. 40 dB HL
   c. 60 dB HL
   d. 80 dB HL

9. The auditory-verbal method of training children who have hearing impairments
   a. insists on auditory cues exclusively
   b. insists on visual cues exclusively
   c. combines visual with auditory cues
   d. none of the above

10. Public Law 94-142 mandates that
    a. all handicapped children must be educated in regular classrooms
    b. all children who have hearing impairments must be educated in regular classrooms
    c. all children must be educated in the least restrictive environment
    d. children with hearing losses greater than 90 dB HL must be educated in special classrooms

11. The Auditory Global Method states that
    a. the exclusive teaching channel should be auditory
    b. the primary teaching channel should be auditory
    c. the primary teaching channel should be visual
    d. the same teaching methods should be used all over the world

12. Many experts feel that integration of a child with hearing impairment into a regular classroom is best achieved with a teaching method involving
    a. finger spelling
    b. signing
    c. auditory-oral
    d. none of the above

13. The intelligence of young children who have severe hearing impairments is best determined by tests that
    a. rely heavily on language
    b. rely lightly on language
    c. rely heavily on performance
    d. include finger spelling for instruction

14. Assessing personality in young children who cannot hear is difficult because
    a. tests are complicated by vocabulary items
    b. personality development is related closely to language development
    c. emotional immaturity is caused by frustration in some children
    d. all of the above

15. Teaching children who cannot hear to speak involves senses that are
    a. tactile
    b. kinesthetic
    c. visual
    d. all of the above

16. Children who are prelinguistically hearing impaired are not those who
    a. lose hearing shortly after birth
    b. are born with hearing loss
    c. lose hearing before they learn language
    d. lose hearing after they learn language

17. Teaching systems for children who cannot hear that include vision, hearing, tactile, and kinesthetic senses are called
    a. unisensory
    b. auditory verbal
    c. multisensory
    d. ASL
18. Auditory training may take advantage of
    a. a wearable hearing aid
    b. a magnetic loop system
    c. an FM carrier system
    d. all of the above
19. Speechreading is usually taught to children
    a. in isolation
    b. in combination with other lessons
    c. without amplification
    d. in darkened areas to increase concentration
20. Many experts agree that children with hearing losses sufficient to require hearing aids should be fitted
    a. when the child can care for the instruments
    b. at the age when children normally begin to speak
    c. at the earliest possible time regardless of age
    d. when the child reaches school age

Answers—Unit B

Matching	*Outline*	*Multiple Choice*
1. a	**1.** E	**1.** a
2. f	**2.** G	**2.** c
3. e	**3.** H	**3.** b
4. h	**4.** O	**4.** b
5. c	**5.** R	**5.** a
6. i	**6.** D	**6.** d
7. b	**7.** I	**7.** d
8. g	**8.** K	**8.** d
9. d	**9.** N	**9.** a
	10. C	**10.** c
	11. J	**11.** b
	12. S	**12.** c
	13. T	**13.** c
	14. A	**14.** d
	15. B	**15.** d
	16. F	**16.** d
	17. L	**17.** c
	18. M	**18.** d
	19. P	**19.** b
	20. Q	**20.** c
	21. U	
	22. V	

PART II

Case Studies

1

History

Your patient is a 26-year-old female with a complaint of diminished hearing "for several years," that "seems to be getting worse." Her mother has told her that she experienced ear infections as a small child, but the patient herself has no memory of this. She has increased difficulty hearing while chewing but seems, to her surprise, to understand speech better in a noisy background than in quiet places. The patient has two older sisters with hearing losses that began in early adulthood. One wears hearing aids successfully and the other was helped by surgery, the nature of which the patient does not know. She, along with members of her family, has a bluish cast to the whites of her eyes. Given the audiometric data on the following page and this history, make your diagnosis and substantiate it.

Diagnosis

Type of Loss   *Right:* _____   *Left:* _____

Probable Etiology

_____

Case Management

_____

_____

_____

_____

_____

Reasons for Decision

_____

_____

_____

_____

Audiometric Data

Test	Right Ear	Left Ear
SRT	25 dB HL	35 dB HL
WRS	98%	100%
ARTs (ipsilateral)	Absent	Absent
ARTs (contralateral)	Absent	Absent
Static compliance	0.7 cc	0.65 cc
ABR	All waves prolonged; interpeak latencies normal; latency-intensity function normal	All waves prolonged; interpeak latencies normal; latency-intensity function normal
TEOAE	Absent	Absent
SISI at 4000 Hz	0%	5%
Tone decay test	0 dB of decay in 60 seconds	5 dB of decay in 60 seconds

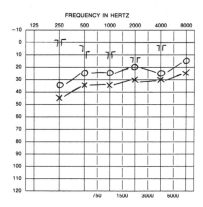

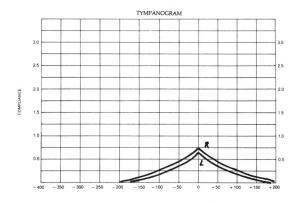

Correct Diagnosis

Type of Loss
Right: Conductive
Left: Conductive

Probable Etiology
Bilateral otosclerosis

Case Management
Refer to an otologist with a good track record doing stapedectomies. Include all audiometric data and a report stating your suspicions. Request a letter to learn the otologic diagnosis and proposed treatment.

Reasons for Decision
The normal bone conduction, air-bone gaps, and excellent word recognition scores all indicate a conductive hearing loss. The tympanograms are Type A in both ears, and crossed and uncrossed acoustic reflexes are absent at the limits of the equipment, suggesting middle-ear disorders. Static compliance is normal and does not assist in diagnosis. The low-frequency tilt of the audiogram suggests stiffness in the middle-ear system. The Carhart notch suggests otosclerosis, along with the family history of females with progressive hearing loss, blue sclera, paracusis willisii, and deprecusis. All special tests are consistent with a conductive hearing loss. The infections as a child have no bearing because the hearing loss had its onset years after the infections had ceased. Because one sister was helped by surgery and the other did well with hearing aids (suggesting good speech recognition ability), it is likely that they too have otosclerosis.

Notes

2

History

Your patient is a 39-year-old male with a history of sudden hearing loss in the right ear and vertigo. Previous to an incident several months earlier, the patient had no difficulty with either hearing or balance. The course of symptoms is described as follows: The patient first noted a sensation of fullness in his right ear along with some slight difficulty understanding through that ear over the telephone. On the second day he noticed a humming noise in that ear followed by a loud roaring sound. He suddenly had the sensation of whirling and was unable to keep his balance; he became ill and vomited several times. He now feels that he has no hearing in his right ear although the spinning sensation has completely disappeared. Both his parents had difficulty hearing when they became much older. His greatest communication difficulty is in group situations or when people speak softly to him on his right side. Given the audiometric findings on the following page and this history, make your diagnosis and substantiate it.

Diagnosis

Type of Loss   Right: _____   Left: _____

Probable Etiology

_____

Case Management

_____
_____
_____
_____
_____

Reasons for Decision

_____
_____
_____
_____

Audiometric Data

Test	Right Ear	Left Ear
SRT	70 dB HL	35 dB HL
WRS	34%	100%
ARTs (ipsilateral)	90 dB HL	100 dB HL
ARTs (contralateral)	95 dB HL	100 dB HL
Static compliance	0.9 cc	0.65 cc
ABR	All waves prolonged; interpeak latencies normal; latency-intensity function for wave V steep	All waves normal; interpeak latencies normal; latency-intensity function for wave V normal
TEOAE	Absent	Present
SISI at 4000 Hz	100%	5%
ABLB	Recruitment	—
Tone decay test	15 dB of decay in 60 seconds	5 dB of decay in 60 seconds

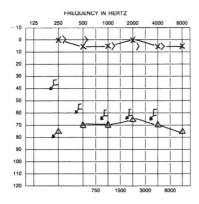

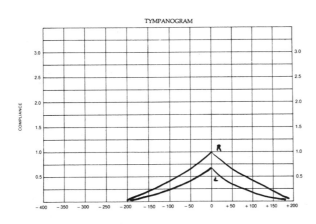

Correct Diagnosis

Type of Loss
Right: Sensorineural (Cochlear)
Left: Normal hearing

Probable Etiology
Unilateral Méniére disease

Case Management
Refer to an otologist with comments on your suspicions and recommend electronystag-mography. If you can perform ENG in your clinic, proceed with the test following your clinic's protocol. Request a report from the physician and arrange for the patient to return for further counseling and longitudinal testing to monitor for fluctuation or progression.

Reasons for Decision
The roaring tinnitus and full aural sensations are part of the usual prodroma of Méniére disease, probably caused by increased endolymphatic pressure. All of the special tests suggest a cochlear site of lesion. The word-recognition score is extremely poor in the right ear. *All* tests in the right ear should have been performed with masking in the left ear. The presence of acoustic reflexes at normal hearing levels (low sensation levels in the right ear), along with the steep ABR latency-intensity function and absent TEOAEs suggests a cochlear disorder. The hearing losses experienced by the patient's parents do not bear on the diagnosis because they are probably caused by aging. The difficulty hearing in groups is typical of severe unilateral losses. Because hearing is normal in the left ear, the patient relies on it and is unaware of the residual hearing in the right ear.

Notes

History

Your patient is a 34-month-old male who is brought to you by his parents. They are not certain whether a hearing loss is present, although the child says "huh" a good deal. The father believes that he "does not pay attention." The child has been "slightly behind" his two older, normal siblings (a boy and a girl) in his language development milestones. A pediatrician has treated the child with antibiotics for "ear infections" on a few occasions, but more often for "tonsillitis." No marked temperature elevations were associated with these episodes, and the child is otherwise healthy. There is no family history of hearing loss, although his father has difficulty understanding speech in groups and has a constant high-pitched tinnitus since serving two years in the artillery. The child tired quickly before all the desired hearing tests could be completed, but given the history and the limited audiometric data on the following page, make your diagnosis and substantiate it.

Diagnosis

Type of Loss   *Right:* _____   *Left:* _____

Probable Etiology

_____

Case Management

_____
_____
_____
_____
_____

Reasons for Decision

_____
_____
_____
_____

Audiometric Data

Test	Right Ear	Left Ear
SRT	20 dB HL	25 dB HL
WRS	?	?
ARTs (ipsilateral)	Absent	Absent
ARTs (contralateral)	Absent	Absent
Static compliance	0.25 cc	0.20 cc
ABR	All waves prolonged; interpeak latencies normal; latency-intensity function normal	All waves prolonged; interpeak latencies normal; latency-intensity function normal
TEOAE	Absent	Absent

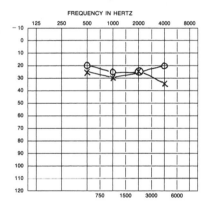

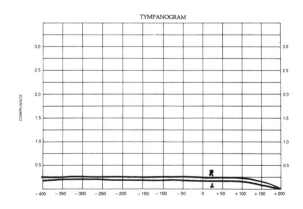

Correct Diagnosis

Type of Loss
Right: Conductive
Left: Conductive

Probable Etiology
Bilateral serous effusion

Case Management
Refer to an otologist with all your findings and suspicions. Make an appointment for further audiometric study, especially bone conduction. Request a report of the physician's findings. Stress to the parents the importance of a complete audiometric examination after all medical and/or surgical treatment has been completed. If hearing is normal upon the return visit, consider referring to a speech-language pathologist to test for language delay secondary to sensory deprivation. Suggest that the father consider a hearing evaluation for a diagnosis of his hearing problem.

Reasons for Decision
The agreement between the SRT and pure-tone average makes the diagnosis of mild hearing loss likely. The fact that the child did not take the bone-conduction test, and the lack of word-recognition scores, makes it impossible to state with certainty that the hearing loss is purely conductive (hence the need for further testing); however, the Type B tympanogram, the absent acoustic reflexes, low static compliance, and flat audiometric configuration all suggest fluid in the middle ear. Because there was no ear drainage, pain, or fever in the history, it is more likely that the hearing loss is due to serous effusion than to active infection. This, of course, must be determined medically. The father's hearing loss is acquired, probably because of noise, and is irrelevant to the diagnosis of the child's problem.

Notes

History

Your patient is a 23-year-old male who was referred by his attorney for routine hearing tests because of a gradual hearing loss in his left ear associated with noise. The patient is a construction worker. There is no history of ear infections, vertigo, or tinnitus, and no reported family members with hearing loss. The patient claims that he is "totally deaf" in the left ear and requests that you write a letter to this effect "to whom it may concern." He claims that he cannot hear people speak at all when they are on his left side. Given the history and the audiometric data on the following page make your diagnosis and substantiate it.

Diagnosis

Type of Loss   *Right:* _____   *Left:* _____

Probable Etiology

_____

Case Management

_____
_____
_____
_____
_____

Reasons for Decision

_____
_____
_____
_____

Audiometric Data

Test	Right Ear	Left Ear
SRT	5 dB HL	NR
WRS	100%	NR
ARTs (ipsilateral)	95 dB HL	95 dB HL
ARTs (contralateral)	100 dB HL	95 dB HL
Static compliance	0.62 cc	0.66 cc
ABR	All waves normal; interpeak latencies normal; latency-intensity function normal	All waves normal; interpeak latencies normal; latency-intensity function normal
TEOAE	Present	Present

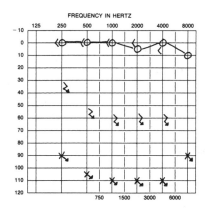

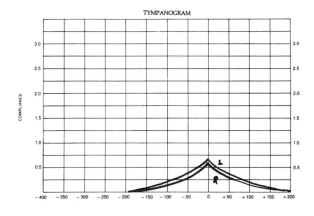

Correct Diagnosis

Type of Loss
Right: Normal hearing
Left: Normal hearing

Probable Etiology
Nonorganic hearing loss (probably malingering)

Case Management
Prepare a report in detail outlining your reasons for suspecting nonorganic hearing loss and the tests that support the diagnosis. Retain and carefully file all test forms or paper read-outs for easy retrieval. Explain to the patient that his test results are inconsistent but that you believe the hearing in his left ear to be normal or near normal. Write a letter to his attorney stating the same thing. Do not use the word "malingering." Suggest reevaluation.

Reasons for Decision
Your suspicions are aroused when the patient claims that he cannot hear people "at all" from the left side. The first audiometric tip-off to nonorganicity was the obvious lack of a shadow curve on the audiogram. If the left ear truly had a total loss, the air-conduction and speech recognition thresholds would have been about 55 dB (average interaural attenuation) and the bone-conduction thresholds no worse than about 15 dB. Word recognition scores obtained at high levels in the "deaf" ear should approach 100 percent as the opposite (normal) ear should respond. The normal levels at which acoustic reflexes were elicited with stimulation to the left ear prove that a total hearing loss is impossible. Further special tests should have been performed as time allowed. High on the list of desirable tests would be the Stenger, using spondaic words and several different frequencies; the pure-tone DAF; and the SPAR test. Existing evidence for nonorganic hearing loss is clear, and malingering is likely because of the involvement of an attorney and potential lawsuit, but psychogenesis cannot be ruled out with certainty. If the hearing loss was truly caused by noise, it would have been less severe and bilateral in nature. Remember that you cannot legally release your findings or impressions to another party without express written permission by the patient.

Notes

History

Your patient is a 42-year-old right-handed male who complains of a high-pitched ringing in his ears, which is louder and more prolonged after noise exposure than had formerly been the case. He is fond of deer and duck hunting and enjoys listening to rock music under earphones. His two sisters have progressive hearing losses that began in their twenties and seemed to get worse during pregnancy. The patient is uncertain whether he has a hearing loss per se but notices that speech often sounds muffled, and he has difficulty hearing in groups or in background noise. He has never had ear infections. Given the history and the audiometric data on the following page make your diagnosis and substantiate it.

Diagnosis

Type of Loss   *Right:* _____   *Left:* _____

Probable Etiology

_____

Case Management

_____
_____
_____
_____
_____

Reasons for Decision

_____
_____
_____
_____

Audiometric Data

Test	Right Ear	Left Ear
SRT	10 dB HL	10 dB HL
WRS	100%	100%
ARTs (ipsilateral)	95 dB HL	90 dB HL
ARTs (contralateral)	95 dB HL	90 dB HL
Static compliance	0.52 cc	0.70 cc
ABR	All waves prolonged; interpeak latencies normal; latency-intensity function steep	All waves prolonged; interpeak latencies normal; latency-intensity function steep
TEOAE	Absent	Absent
SISI at 4000 Hz	100%	100%
Tone decay test	5 dB of decay in 60 seconds	5 dB of decay in 60 seconds

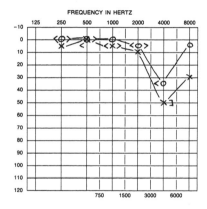

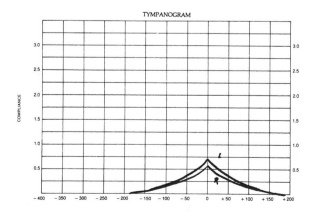

Correct Diagnosis

Type of Loss
Right: Sensorineural (cochlear)
Left: Sensorineural (cochlear)

Probable Etiology
Exposure to high noise levels

Case Management
Explain to the patient the nature of the loss and why the cause is probably noise. Encourage abstention from or minimizing exposure to noise. Suggest the use of hearing protectors, possibly in the form of special impact-noise plugs. If possible, fit the plugs yourself and/or provide the patient with precise information on where foam plugs can be obtained and their approximate cost. Encourage lower levels when listening to music and the use of loudspeakers rather than earphones. Arrange for reevaluation of hearing in six months and stress the importance of checking for progression of the loss. Interoctave frequencies (3000 and 6000 Hz) should have been tested because of the greater-than-20 dB differences in thresholds at octave points.

Reasons for Decision
The audiogram shows the typical acoustic trauma notch; note that the loss at 4000 Hz is greater in the left ear, which is typical of persons firing a rifle from the right shoulder. The family history sounds like otosclerosis, although you cannot be certain of that, but it is unrelated to the patient's problem. It is likely that the patient experiences some increased loss of hearing and tinnitus immediately after noise exposure, both of which had been recovering to a greater extent in the past until the threshold shifts became more permanent. It is also likely that the patient himself realizes that noise is a probable cause of his difficulty, based on his own subjective impressions and his history.

Notes

History

Your patient is a 16-year-old female with a lifelong history of ear infections. She reports having had mastoidectomies on both sides. A strong pungent odor is noticeable near her ears. There is no family history of hearing loss. She claims that her hearing fluctuates, at times appearing to be near normal and at other times creating severe problems in communication. She has tried a hearing aid in her right ear but constant drainage made its use impossible. She has since lost the aid. Her family doctor has told her that nothing can be done to improve her hearing and has her on a renewable prescription for ear drops. Given the case history and the audiometric data on the following page, make your diagnosis and substantiate it.

Diagnosis

Type of Loss   Right: _____   Left: _____

Probable Etiology

_____

Case Management

_____
_____
_____
_____

Reasons for Decision

_____
_____
_____
_____

Audiometric Data

Test	Right Ear	Left Ear
SRT	45 dB HL	40 dB HL
WRS	92%	94%
ARTs (ipsilateral)	Untestable	Untestable
ARTs (contralateral)	Untestable	Untestable
Static compliance	No seal	No seal
ABR	All waves prolonged; interpeak latencies normal; latency-intensity function normal	All waves prolonged; interpeak latencies normal; latency-intensity function normal
TEOAE	Absent	Absent
SISI at 4000 Hz	90%	90%
Tone decay test	0 dB of decay in 60 seconds	5 dB of decay in 60 seconds

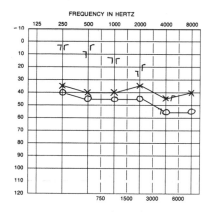

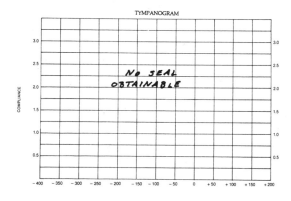

Correct Diagnosis

Type of Loss
Right: Mixed
Left: Mixed

Probable Etiology
Chronic otitis media

Case Management
Discuss with the patient the type of hearing loss she has and its relationship to her history of infections and strongly suggest that she consider a second opinion by an otologist. Provide a detailed report to the otologist and request a letter with his or her diagnosis and plan for therapy. Discuss the possibility of hearing aids if there is no evidence that treatment will result in improvement in hearing. Obtain written medical clearance before proceeding with a hearing-aid evaluation and, if the ear drainage is a persistent problem, consider a bone-conduction aid. Arrange for periodic monitoring of the hearing loss and keep the patient informed of her progress. See that the patient understands the implications of the sensorineural portion of her hearing loss and recognizes that, although her hearing may be improved considerably, it cannot be made completely normal.

Reasons for Decision
The air-bone gap, high word-recognition scores, and drop in bone-conduction sensitivity in the high frequencies all indicate a mixed loss that is predominantly conductive. The cochlear reserve may actually be better than the bone-conduction thresholds indicate because of alterations in the inertial mode of bone conduction caused by the middle-ear disorder, although the high SISI scores at 4000 Hz indicate sensorineural involvement. If tested, auditory evoked potentials and otoacoustic emissions would be consistent with the cochlear portion of the hearing loss. The inability to obtain a seal upon immittance testing and the large C_1 values suggest tympanic membrane perforations, which should have been visible upon otoscopic examination prior to testing. The strong odor at the ears suggests the possibility of cholesteatomas. Diplomacy is necessary in making the new referral so that your comments will not be construed as critical of the family doctor, although surely this consultation may be necessary.

Notes

History

Your patient is a 51-year-old male who complains of vague difficulty in understanding speech, especially in noisy or otherwise untoward listening circumstances. He has no history of ear disease, skull trauma, balance difficulties, or noise exposure. Sometimes he feels that his understanding is improved if he pays very close attention. He has been seen for medical examination and no explanation for his difficulty was offered, although you are not certain of the extent of this examination. Given the history and the audiometric data on the following page, make your diagnosis and substantiate it.

Diagnosis

Type of Loss   Right: _____   Left: _____

Probable Etiology

_____

Case Management

_____

_____

_____

_____

_____

Reasons for Decision

_____

_____

_____

_____

Audiometric Data

Test	Right Ear	Left Ear
SRT	0 dB HL	5 dB HL
WRS	98%	100%
ARTs (ipsilateral)	85 dB HL	90 dB HL
ARTs (contralateral)	Absent	Absent
Static compliance	0.72 cc	0.80 cc
ABR	All waves prolonged; interpeak latencies normal; latency-intensity function normal	All waves prolonged; interpeak latencies normal; latency-intensity function normal
TEOAE	Present	Present
SISI at 4000 Hz	0%	5%
Tone decay test	0 dB of decay in 60 seconds	5 dB of decay in 60 seconds

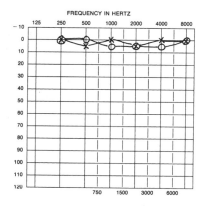

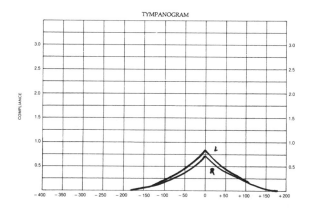

Correct Diagnosis

Type of Loss
Right: Normal sensitivity
Left: Normal sensitivity

Probable Etiology
Unknown; possible brainstem lesion

Case Management
Reschedule the patient for a complete battery of special tests for central auditory disorders to include AMLR, PI-PB functions, SSI-ICM, SSI-CCM, staggered spondaic words, and others available. Tell the patient that his difficulty is not in sounds being loud enough because the audiogram indicates normal hearing for pure tones. Explain that additional stress will have to be placed on his word recognition ability to determine the extent of his difficulty beyond what can be derived from testing with standard word lists. Discuss referral to a neurologist, which would best be done after additional audiometric studies have been completed.

Reasons for Decision
The normal hearing sensitivity, with the kinds of complaints the patient makes, alerts you to a possible central disorder. Present ipsilateral acoustic reflexes at normal levels indicate normal middle ears and acoustic pathways, including VIIth nerve integrity, short of the crossover pathways in the brainstem. Absent contralateral acoustic reflexes suggest that the crossover pathways are involved. Low scores on the modified SISI also suggest a central lesion. More definitive testing should help in the diagnosis, but a neurological referral is imperative in any case.

Notes

CASE

8

History

Your patient is a 19-year-old female college student. Her main complaint is a hearing loss that presents more difficulty in hearing and understanding speech than in hearing environmental sounds. She has had this difficulty as long as she can remember and does not believe it is getting worse. There are no known family members with a hearing loss, and she has never had any ear infections, nor has she worn hearing aids. The patient's speech is quite intelligible but there is some distortion in the production of her sibilant sounds, and her vocal tone is rather monotonous. She managed to get good grades in high school, but now that she is in college, she finds school much more difficult and believes it is because of her hearing problem. You notice that she speaks rather loudly. Given the history and the audiometric data on the following page make your diagnosis and substantiate it.

Diagnosis

Type of Loss   *Right:* _____   *Left:* _____

Probable Etiology

_____

Case Management

_____
_____
_____
_____

Reasons for Decision

_____
_____
_____
_____

Audiometric Data

Test	Right Ear	Left Ear
SRT	45 dB HL	40 dB HL
WRS	86%	82%
ARTs (ipsilateral)	90 dB HL	95 dB HL
ARTs (contralateral)	90 dB HL	90 dB HL
Static compliance	0.80 cc	0.78 cc
ABR	All waves prolonged; interpeak latencies normal; latency-intensity function steep	All waves prolonged; interpeak latencies normal; latency-intensity function steep
TEOAE	Absent	Absent
SISI at 4000 Hz	100%	100%
Tone decay test	10 dB of decay in 60 seconds	15 dB of decay in 60 seconds

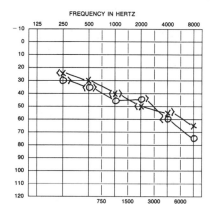

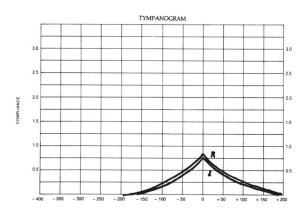

Correct Diagnosis

Type of Loss
Right: Sensorineural (probably cochlear)
Left: Sensorineural (probably cochlear)

Probable Etiology
Unknown; possibly congenital

Case Management
Discuss with the patient the possibility of a hearing-aid evaluation, trial period with hearing aids, and a period of auditory rehabilitation and hearing-aid orientation. Ascertain that the patient understands the nature of her hearing loss. Arrange for medical consultation prior to making ear impressions, if this is required in your state. Try to make a positive yet realistic appraisal of the patient's potential for hearing-aid use. If she wishes medical consultation on the irreversibility of her hearing loss, offer to provide your findings to the physician of her choice. Check with the physician on possible blood studies and inquire about her interest in genetic counseling. If she is not interested in audiological rehabilitation at this time, recommend that she have annual reevaluations of her hearing.

Reasons for Decision
The absent air-bone gaps and diminished word-recognition scores, along with the normal tympanograms, indicate sensorineural hearing loss. The low sensation level acoustic reflexes and high SISI scores suggest a cochlear site of lesion. There is simply not enough information in the history to hazard more than a guess about the cause of the loss. The fact that the patient does not know of family members with hereditary hearing loss does not mean that there have been none. The loss may also have been acquired at an early age, caused by some disease.

Notes

History

Your patient is a 58-year-old female with a complaint of hearing loss in her right ear. The difficulty was first noticed about five years earlier and has been gradually progressive to the point where she relies entirely on her left ear for communication . She does not experience true vertigo, but frequently she has attacks of unsteadiness and occasional headaches. She also complains of a constant noise in her right ear, which she describes as "bacon frying." Her family physician has told her that the hearing loss is related to several episodes of middle-ear infection that she had as a child. Her main communication problem is in groups or noisy backgrounds, which she attempts to avoid. Given this history and the audiometric data on the following page, make your diagnosis and substantiate it.

Diagnosis

Type of Loss   *Right:* _____   *Left:* _____

Probable Etiology

_____

Case Management

_____
_____
_____
_____
_____

Reasons for Decision

_____
_____
_____
_____

Audiometric Data

Test	Right Ear	Left Ear
SRT	50 dB HL	5 dB HL
WRS	6%	100%
ARTs (ipsilateral)	Absent	85 dB HL
ARTs (contralateral)	Absent	80 dB HL
Static compliance	0.80 cc	0.83 cc
ABR	All waves prolonged; interpeak latencies normal; latency-intensity function shallow	All waves normal; interpeak latencies normal; latency-intensity function normal
TEOAE	Present	Present
ABLB	Decruitment	—
Modified SISI at 4000 Hz	0%	100%
Tone decay test	30+ dB of decay in 60 seconds	5 dB of decay in 60 seconds

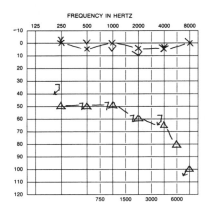

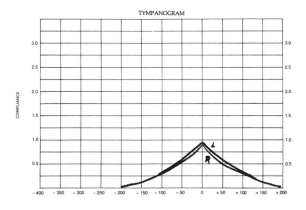

Correct Diagnosis

Type of Loss
Right: Sensorineural (probably neural)
Left: Normal

Probable Etiology
Acoustic neuroma—right side

Case Management
Make a prompt referral, if possible, to a neuro-otologist or to an otologist with experience in dealing with neural lesions in the auditory tract. Detail all your findings and advise him or her that the history and auditory findings are consistent with a possible retrocochlear lesion. You may discuss your impressions of a possible lesion of the VIIIth nerve with the patient, but you should hesitate to put it into a report that is leaving your clinic. Short of frightening the patient, do all you can to see that the referral is followed through. Request that the physician send you results of his or her diagnostic tests (e.g., ENG and radiologic studies), along with the diagnosis and proposed treatment.

Reasons for Decision
The left ear is completely normal on all tests and the right ear shows a moderate loss by both air and bone conduction. SRTs agree nicely with the pure-tone averages, but the word-recognition scores are extremely poor in the right ear for a moderate loss and first raise suspicions of a retrocochlear lesion. The tinnitus is also not of the usual variety described by patients with cochlear pathology. Abnormal ABRs, present TEOAEs, loudness recruitment, marked tone decay, and negative SISI scores all fit with a neural lesion in the right ear. The gradual progressive nature of the loss, the type of dizziness, and the headaches all call for an immediate referral to confirm or deny the presence of a space-occupying lesion. The history of ear infections is unrelated to the present hearing loss.

Notes

10

History

Your patient is an 82-year-old man with a history of gradually progressive hearing loss in both ears over the past fifteen years. He is brought, reluctantly, to the clinic by his daughter-in-law, who complains privately that "he does not pay attention." He claims that sometimes he hears better than at other times and compliments you on the fact that you are easier to understand than most people. He has tried several hearing aids, which were useless to him; he has no desire to purchase any more hearing aids. Because he finds listening in groups difficult, he has ceased attending church, parties, and the theater. He claims that people do not speak clearly and that he understands better when they speak more slowly. Given the history and the audiometric data on the following page, make your diagnosis and substantiate it.

Diagnosis

Type of Loss   *Right:* _____   *Left:* _____

Probable Etiology

_____

Case Management

_____

_____

_____

_____

Reasons for Decision

_____

_____

_____

_____

Audiometric Data

Test	Right Ear	Left Ear
SRT	50 dB HL	45 dB HL
WRS	62%	58%
ARTs (ipsilateral)	95 dB HL	95 dB HL
ARTs (contralateral)	90 dB HL	100 dB HL
Static compliance	0.92 cc	0.65 cc
ABR	All waves prolonged; interpeak latencies normal; latency-intensity function steep	All waves prolonged; interpeak latencies normal; latency-intensity function steep
TEOAE	Absent	Absent
SISI at 4000 Hz	90%	85%
Tone decay test	10 dB of decay in 60 seconds	15 dB of decay in 60 seconds

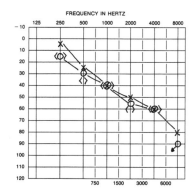

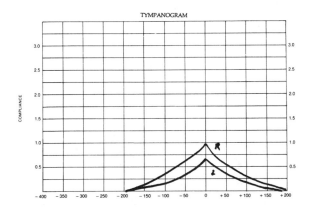

Correct Diagnosis

Type of Loss
Right: Sensorineural
Left: Sensorineural

Probable Etiology
Presbycusis

Case Management
Discuss the possibility of amplification for a trial period. In counseling the family, make sure that you speak directly to the patient, although the daughter-in-law should be present. Listen carefully to his complaints and do not provide more information on the nature of the hearing loss than the patient seems to desire. Advise the family that hearing aids should be purchased on a trial basis until it has been demonstrated that they are of value, and that this cannot really be achieved unless the patient enrolls for a period of auditory rehabilitation that emphasizes coping strategies. Suggest the possibility of assistive listening devices, such as a personal FM system, TV hookup, and telephone amplifier. Be as reassuring as possible, short of making an unethical guarantee that the hearing loss will not progress significantly. Arrange for periodic reevaluations and, if the patient agrees, for earmold fabrication. If state law requires medical concurrence before proceeding, explain this to the family and assist in the arrangements.

Reasons for Decision
All immittance and audiometric results rule out any conductive hearing loss. The lack of an air-bone gap and the relatively poor word recognition all fit with a diagnosis of sensorineural hearing loss. Note that the SRT is slightly poorer than the pure-tone average; this is observed in many elderly patients. Since there is nothing specific in the history to suggest a cause for the hearing loss, it is likely that the patient's advanced age is the etiologic factor. Improved understanding of slower speech, sometimes called "phonemic regression," is sometimes seen in patients with presbycusis. Convincing the patient to give hearing aids one more try will not be easy and should not be approached strenuously. This may come about if the patient feels a sense of confidence in you as an audiologist, or if enrolled in coping strategies classes even without hearing aids.

Notes

11

History

Your patient is a 39-year-old female who complains of a sudden hearing loss following an automobile accident in which her car was struck from the rear. She also claims dizziness, severe bitemporal headaches, nausea, and "blackout spells." She did not mention tinnitus until asked about it during the history taking. There is no reported family history of hearing loss, ear infections, or other symptoms that the patient now claims to experience. She requests that a written report of your findings be sent to her for her records.

Diagnosis

Type of Loss   Right: _____   Left: _____

Probable Etiology

_____

Case Management

_____
_____
_____
_____
_____

Reasons for Decision

_____
_____
_____
_____

Audiometric Data

Test	Right Ear	Left Ear
SRT	30 dB HL	35 dB HL
WRS	86%	80%
ARTs (ipsilateral)	85 dB HL	85 dB HL
ARTs (contralateral)	80 dB HL	85 dB HL
Static compliance	0.70 cc	0.73 cc
ABR	All waves normal; interpeak latencies normal; latency-intensity function normal	All waves normal; interpeak latencies normal; latency-intensity function normal
ABR Wave V threshold	15 dB NHL	20 dB NHL
TEQAE	Present	Present

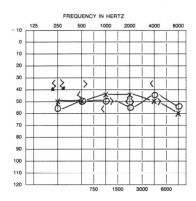

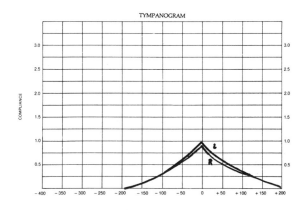

Correct Diagnosis

Type of Loss
Right: Nonorganic hearing loss
Left: Nonorganic hearing loss

Probable Etiology
Possible malingering

Case Management
Complete as many tests for nonorganic hearing loss as time allows. Counsel the patient regarding her inconsistencies and accept the responsibility yourself for not having properly instructed her in taking the tests. Readminister the audiogram and SRT tests if time permits and arrange for rescheduling. Record all your findings in a report and file carefully. Do not confront the patient or act accusatory in any way. State in a separate report to her that inconsistencies preclude diagnosis and do not mention special tests for nonorganic hearing loss.

Reasons for Decision
The main indicator of nonorganicity in this case is the obvious discrepancy between the SRT and the pure-tone average for each ear (the former obtained at considerably lower hearing levels) and the normal acoustic reflexes. Normal ABR results and present TEOAEs suggest normal hearing in both ears. The history itself should have alerted you to possible nonorganicity since the patient may wish to bring suit for damages against the owner of the car that struck hers, but this is not evidence in itself. The primary behavioral tests for you to perform if you so desire, are pure-tone delayed auditory feedback and ascending-descending threshold exploration.

Notes

History

Your patient is a 7-year-old female who failed the public school hearing screenings on two occasions. The child's parents have had her examined by an otologist, who could find no explanation for the apparent high-frequency hearing loss and has referred her to you for further study. The child denies any difficulty in hearing.

Diagnosis

Type of Loss   *Right:* _____   *Left:* _____

Probable Etiology

_____

Case Management

_____

_____

_____

_____

_____

Reasons for Decision

_____

_____

_____

_____

Audiometric Data

Test	Right Ear	Left Ear
SRT	15 dB HL	20 dB HL
WRS	100%	100%
ARTs (ipsilateral)	90 dB HL	90 dB HL
ARTs (contralateral)	100 dB HL	100 dB HL
Static compliance	0.62 cc	0.59 cc
ABR	All waves normal; interpeak latencies normal; latency-intensity function normal	All waves normal; interpeak latencies normal; latency-intensity function normal
TEOAE	Present	Present

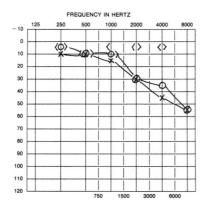

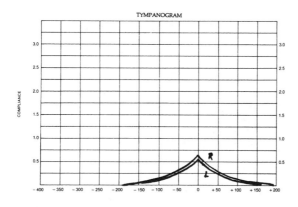

Correct Diagnosis

Type of Loss
Right: Normal hearing
Left: Normal hearing

Probable Etiology
Collapsing ear canals

Case Management
Retest the child with insert receivers, stock earmolds, or plastic tubing in the ear canal to keep the canal open. If normal hearing is demonstrated, explain to the parents what has occurred and that failing the hearing test was no fault of the child. You may demonstrate to the parents how the canal collapses by placing an empty earphone cushion over the ear and allowing them to see the effect of ear canal closure through the opening. Send a letter to the referring physician with the correct audiogram and explanation of your findings.

Reasons for Decision
The high-frequency conductive hearing loss first seen in the absence of positive otological findings and the presence of normal tympanograms and acoustic reflexes are the main indications of collapsing ear canals. It is fairly easy to guess what happened in this case, but the same phenomenon can occur in the presence of a hearing loss, making diagnosis quite obscure. Careful examination at the time of otoscopy, preceding immittance measures, should alert you to possible collapsing canals. ABR and TEOAE results using insert earphones assist in the diagnosis of normal hearing but would probably not have been indicated in routine practice. This case gives testimony to the value of insert receivers. The supra-aural earphones used in the evaluation and in the previous school screenings created external ear canal collapse and false positive findings.

Notes

13

History

Your patient is a 16-year-old male who has had a hearing loss since early childhood when he became very ill with bacterial meningitis. He was educated in schools for deaf children using a manual approach, although he does have some speech. Use of amplification systems such as hearing aids and FM systems have consistently been unsuccessful. Recently, his hearing was evaluated in the office of an otolaryngologist, who diagnosed a severe mixed hearing loss and recommended either exploratory middle-ear surgery (due to the air-bone gaps) or powerful hearing aids.

Diagnosis

Type of Loss   *Right:* _____   *Left:* _____

Probable Etiology

_____

Case Management

_____

_____

_____

_____

_____

Reasons for Decision

_____

_____

_____

_____

Audiometric Data

Test	Right Ear	Left Ear
SRT	NR	NR
WRS	Did not test	Did not test
ARTs (ipsilateral)	Absent	Absent
ARTs (contralateral)	Absent	Absent
Static compliance	0.60 cc	0.57 cc
ABR	NR	NR
TEOAE	Absent	Absent

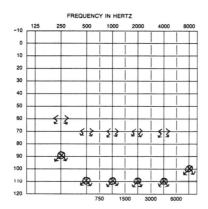

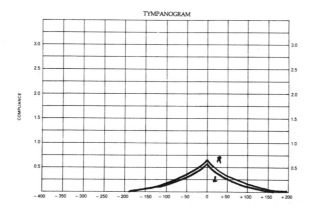

Correct Diagnosis

Type of Loss
Right: Profound sensorineural hearing loss
Left: Profound sensorineural hearing loss

Probable Etiology
Severe cochlear damage due to childhood meningitis

Case Management
Retesting the patient with insert receivers instead of standard supra-aural phones results in no responses at the maximum limits of the audiometer. Moving the bone-conduction oscillator from the forehead to the mastoid process results in disappearance of the bone-conduction responses. These factors suggest that all the original responses were vibrotactile rather than auditory. Suggestion should be made to the physician that the apparent air-bone gap is false, obviating middle-ear surgery, and that the total lack of response by air conduction makes successful use of hearing aids unlikely. The possibility of a cochlear implant may be pursued, as well as vibrotactile devices, but the family should be made aware of the limitations this may have considering the boy's systems of communication.

Reasons for Decision
The responses originally obtained near the limit of the audiometric equipment for air and bone conduction suggested the possibility of vibrotactile responses. The air-conduction responses disappeared with the use of insert receivers since they do not mechanically vibrate the skull to the extent that supra-aural receivers do. The reason that the bone-conduction threshold became higher when the oscillator was moved to the mastoid was that tactile responses are known to require more intensity from the mastoid than from the forehead, and auditory responses require less intensity from the mastoid than from the forehead. Attempts at changing the patient's system of communication should be approached thoughtfully considering his history.

Notes

History

Your patient is a 79-year-old male, who has had a gradually progressive bilateral hearing loss for about fifteen years. He denies a history of ear infections or noise exposure. He experiences his greatest difficulties in discriminating speech in the presence of background noise. His main complaint is a sudden drooping of the right side of his face, which he attributes to a severe cold several days earlier. He says he thinks the paralysis may be "getting better." He states at the outset that he has no interest in purchasing hearing aids.

Diagnosis

Type of Loss *Right:* _____ *Left:* _____

Probable Etiology

_____

Case Management

_____
_____
_____
_____
_____

Reasons for Decision

_____
_____
_____
_____

Audiometric Data

Test	Right Ear	Left Ear
SRT	15 dB HL	15 dB HL
WRS	88%	84%
ARTs (ipsilateral)	Absent	95 dB HL
ARTs (contralateral)	90 dB HL	Absent
Static compliance	0.50 cc	0.54 cc
ABR	All waves prolonged; interpeak latencies normal; latency-intensity function steep	All waves prolonged; interpeak latencies normal; latency-intensity function steep
TEOAE	Present	Present
SISI at 4000 Hz	100%	100%
Tone decay test at 4000 Hz	10 dB of decay in 60 seconds	15 dB of decay in 60 seconds

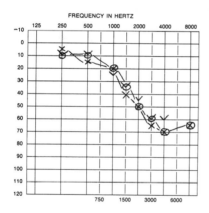

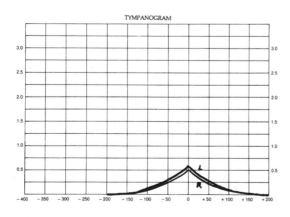

Correct Diagnosis

Type of Loss
Right: Mild cochlear hearing loss
Left: Mild cochlear hearing loss

Probable Etiology
Presbycusis
VIIth cranial nerve damage (right).
Probably Bell's palsy

Case Management
Discuss the use of hearing aids without overstressing their potential value. Suggest that the patient see an otolaryngologist because of the facial palsy. Be as reassuring as possible without promising complete remission of the paralysis. Suggest retesting his hearing in one year, or sooner if he notices any change.

Reasons for Decision
The history and audiological findings are consistent with a cochlear lesion and, given the history, is most likely produced by aging. The probability of Bell's palsy on the right side is suggested by the history of sudden onset, the trend toward spontaneous improvement, and because of the lack of ipsilateral and contralateral acoustic reflexes when the probe assembly of the immittance device is placed in the right ear (involving the right facial nerve). The facial paralysis is unrelated to the hearing loss.

Notes

History

Your patient is a 28-year-old female who complains of disturbing difficulties comprehending conversations within background noise. She states that she has trouble engaging in social interactions at parties, family gatherings, sporting events, and similar environments where noise levels are high. She reports that others seem to have little or no difficulty in these situations and that friends have begun to question her hearing abilities. In quieter listening environments she reports no difficulties. She has no history of ear infections, vertigo, or tinnitus, and reports no current or past employment or recreational noise exposure. There is no reported history of hearing loss in her family. Given the history and the audiometric data on the following page make your diagnosis and substantiate it.

Diagnosis

Type of Loss   Right: _____   Left: _____

Probable Etiology

_____

Case Management

_____
_____
_____
_____
_____

Reasons for Decision

_____
_____
_____
_____

Audiometric Data

Test	Right Ear	Left Ear
SRT	0 dB HL	5 dB HL
WRS	96%	100%
ARTs (ipsilateral)	90 dB HL	95 dB HL
ARTs (contralateral)	90 dB HL	90 dB HL
Static compliance	0.35 cc	1.15 cc
ABR	All waves normal; interpeak latencies normal; latency-intensity function normal	All waves normal; interpeak latencies normal; latency-intensity function normal
TEOAE	Present	Present

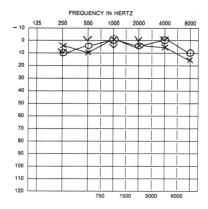

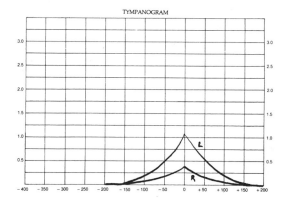

Correct Diagnosis

Type of Loss
Right: Normal hearing
Left: Normal hearing

Probable Etiology
Obscure auditory dysfunction

Case Management
Discuss the normal test findings with the patient. Explain that while the underlying reason for her expressed difficulties is not always identifiable, that does not diminish the reality of the difficulties she is experiencing in social contexts. Having ruled out peripheral auditory dysfunction, outline possible underlying explanations for the difficulties, including anxiety or mild auditory processing problems surfacing only when listening conditions are more taxing. Offer to make referral for further evaluation of these possibilities if desired. Otherwise, in the absence of identifiable peripheral hearing disorder, treat the complaints as stemming from the basis of a situational hearing loss, providing counseling on communication strategies, employment of assistive listening devices, and possible alterations in environmental/listening settings. Recommend a follow-up evaluation in one year, or sooner, if additional symptoms develop.

Reasons for Decision
The normal results for all tests rules out the presence of peripheral auditory pathology. The complaints presented by this patient are real and need to be addressed proactively in an effort to decrease their impact. Given the usual desire of patients to uncover etiology whenever possible, the discussion of potential etiologies and the offered referral for further evaluation is indicated.

Notes

$50 = 10 \log (\quad)$

$- 10 [\quad 5 \quad]$

$\log (\quad) = 5$ $\qquad 100,000 = 10^{+5}$

$\dfrac{10^{-7}}{10^{-12}}$ $\qquad 10^{-11} \quad ^{-7 + 16 =}$ $\qquad '$

$-7k + 12 = \quad +5$

$\dfrac{200}{20} = 100$

$\log = 2$

$100 \times 2 = 200$